"A compassionate and inclusive look at the impact of the Zika epidemic: from the mothers of affected babies to the race for an effective treatment."

Laura Rodrigues, London School of
Hygiene & Tropical Medicine

"Ingeniously crafted and affectingly narrated, *Zika* is a momentous contribution to the critical study of science and global health."

João Biehl, Princeton University

"Diniz illustrates the devastating effects that Zika's spread has had on impoverished women, and how government scientists and policy makers failed to live up to their responsibilities toward those affected. A brilliant read, highly recommended!"

Udo Schuklenk, Queen's University, Canada

# ZIKA

## FROM THE BRAZILIAN BACKLANDS TO GLOBAL THREAT

## DEBORA DINIZ

Translated by
Diane Grosklaus Whitty

ZED

*Zika: From the Brazilian Backlands to Global Threat* was first published in English in 2017 by Zed Books Ltd, The Foundry, 17 Oval Way, London SE11 5RR, UK.

www.zedbooks.net

First published in Brazil by Civilização Brasileria
Rights for this edition negotiated via Seibel Publishing Services Ltd.

Typeset in Adobe Caslon Pro and Eurostile-Condensed by Swales & Willis Ltd, Exeter, Devon
Fact checkers: Gabriela Rondon, Luciana Brito, Sinara Gumieri
Librarian: Illy Batista
Cover design by Keith Dodds
Printed and bound by CPI Group (UK) Ltd, Croydon, CR0 4YY

A catalogue record for this book is available from the British Library.

ISBN 978-1-78699-159-1 hb
ISBN 978-1-78699-158-4 pb
ISBN 978-1-78699-160-7 pdf
ISBN 978-1-78699-161-4 epub
ISBN 978-1-78699-162-1 mobi

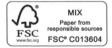

MIX
Paper from responsible sources
FSC
www.fsc.org  FSC® C013604

# CONTENTS

# CONTENTS

# ACKNOWLEDGMENTS

This book bears witness to the first year of the Zika virus epidemic in Brazil. The story was constructed from the oral accounts of dozens of women, doctors, and scientists as well as from Brazilian and international press reports and a vast amount of academic scholarship. I could not have written it in such timely fashion without the assistance of countless individuals – too many to be named in this brief space. All I can say is that you were essential. Thank you. In particular, I am grateful to the doctors and scientists who were so generous in explaining epidemiological and biomedical jargon to me and shedding light on controversies, and who had me watch everything from laboratory procedures to deliveries. All of them manifested a genuine desire to share their stories. I hope I have honored their enormous vote of confidence. I have only one person to thank for the English translation, Diane Grosklaus Whitty, without whom the words and ideas in these pages would have remained entangled in the Brazilian mind. Lastly, I thank every single woman who told me her story, welcomed me into her home, and asked me to write this book so neither she nor her child would be forgotten. I don't know if I managed to accomplish this weighty mission, but here is my promise to tell their story.

# TRANSLATOR'S NOTE

Most of the voices you will hear in these pages belong to people who live in an obscure corner of the world that is generally ignored by the rest of us. Brazil's 2015 Zika epidemic cast them into a temporary spotlight, only to leave behind a trail of destruction. It also left them with a story to tell. Debora Diniz gave these voices a stage in the original Portuguese version of this book and then entrusted me with the task of enabling them to be understood by English readers.

In translation, the question is always how best to accomplish this task. Debora agreed with me that fluency was paramount, so readers could immerse themselves in an unknown culture without feeling like intimidated immigrants struggling to stay afloat. In some cases, this meant adding to the text, for example, providing background on Fiocruz, Brazil's giant public health foundation, or painting a brief portrait of Northeast Brazil, the setting for much of the action. In others, it meant subtracting. For instance, a few side notes and allusions that would easily be understood by Brazilians but require a convoluted explanation for a foreign audience were eliminated. In still other cases, it entailed interpreting more than translating, as when the geographical reference "Alto Sertão, Sertão, and Cariri" (not immediately clear even to most Brazilians outside the Northeast) was simplified to "rural Paraíba." Whether

I was adding, subtracting, or interpreting, the goal was to remove distractions from the narrative itself, and the changes were always made with Debora's agreement and often assistance.

Perhaps most importantly, the linguistic differences between Portuguese and English are not limited to the words or sentence structures in which ideas come cloaked. Narration itself has its own mind in each language. Brazilian readers move effortlessly from historical present to past and then back again, sometimes within one paragraph. Try this in English and your reader will soon be flipping pages, trying to figure out when the action takes place. In weaving a tale where several threads play out simultaneously, Debora could allow herself great leeway in Portuguese, shifting easily not only between verb tenses but also between settings and timeframes. Since the English-speaking mind demands greater linearity, some sections of the book underwent significant re-organization. Again, Debora was in wholehearted agreement about tearing down any barriers between story and audience, and she signed off on all changes.

This is not to say that the book has been stripped of all Brazilianness. Readers will learn of the evil eye, the Feast of St John's day in rural Paraíba, the geographical hierarchy within the Brazilian scientific community. Moreover, the story itself is steeped in the flavor of Brazil, from the way science was done to how people interacted. It is in the realm of these human interactions that readers will find the most foreignized facet of this translation: the characters have retained the names by which they are known in Brazil. Dr Kleber Luz does not become "Dr Luz" or "Luz," as in international press reports, but remains "Dr Kleber." Many of these people shared deeply personal memories with Debora, and I felt that to rename them would somehow be a betrayal of their trust.

In closing, my thanks to my husband Michael, whose insights, linguistic and otherwise, make him my prime sounding board and first reader. Immense thanks as well to Debora, for trusting me to re-tell this story in English. And like the author, I hope my words will do justice to the voices of the women and men portrayed here.

# PRINCIPAL CHARACTERS

## THE MOTHERS

**Géssica Eduardo dos Santos**

Mother of Guilherme, who was born with microcephaly and died shortly after birth, in February 2016. Géssica donated her son's body to research and his baby things to another baby born with microcephaly. She lives in Juazeirinho, in rural Paraíba.

**Maria da Conceição Alcantara Oliveira Matias (Conceição)**

Mother of Catarina Maria, born with microcephaly in February 2016. A physical therapist, Conceição now dedicates herself to providing her daughter with early stimulation. She lives in Juazeirinho, in rural Paraíba.

**Sofia Tezza**

Italian woman who was infected by Zika while pregnant and living in Brazil. Sofia lost her baby in October 2015 and donated him to research. Slovenian scientists found the Zika virus in his body, proof of vertical transmission.

# THE DOCTORS

**Adriana Melo**

Obstetrician from Campina Grande, in rural Paraíba, and specialist in fetal medicine, who drew amniotic fluid from two of her patients, Géssica and Conceição, proof of vertical transmission.

**Antônio Bandeira**

Infectious disease specialist from Salvador, Bahia, who cared for patients stricken by a mysterious new disease in Camaçari.

**Carlos Brito**

General practitioner and epidemiologist from Recife, Pernambuco, whose bedside experience prompted him to suspect that Zika was circulating in Brazil.

**Celso Tavares**

Infectious disease specialist from Maceio, Alagoas, who noticed the first signs of a new disease while caring for patients in the countryside of his state.

**Kleber Luz**

Pediatrician and epidemiologist from Natal, Rio Grande do Norte, who hypothesized that Zika was the new virus circulating in Brazil.

**Melania Amorim**

Obstetrician from Campina Grande, in rural Paraíba, and advocate of humanized childbirth; formerly Dr Adriana's professor and today her close colleague.

## Vanessa and Ana Van der Linden

Mother and daughter neuropediatricians from Recife, Pernambuco, who investigated a surge in cases of babies with microcephaly in the latter half of 2015.

# THE SCIENTISTS

## Ana Bispo

Researcher at Fiocruz, in Rio de Janeiro, who detected the Zika virus in amniotic fluid drawn from Conceição and Géssica in November 2015.

## Cláudia Duarte dos Santos

Virologist at the Oswaldo Cruz Institute (Fiocruz) in southern Brazil, who detected Zika in blood samples received from Dr Kleber.

## Gúbio Soares Campos

Virologist and professor at the Federal University of Bahia. In late April 2016, he and his wife, Silvia Sardi, ran lab tests that identified Zika as the new virus in Brazil.

## Silvia Sardi

Virologist and professor at the Federal University of Bahia. She met her husband, Gúbio Soares, when he was doing his PhD in her native Buenos Aires. In late April 2016, the couple ran lab tests that identified Zika as the new virus in Brazil.

# TIMELINE

### APRIL 29, 2015

A virus that causes a mysterious illness has been detected in Salvador. The symptoms are similar to those of dengue but less serious. Researchers believe the virus reached Brazil during the World Cup.

Online news report, G1, Bahia

### MAY 14, 2015

The Ministry of Health confirmed this Thursday that the Zika virus is circulating in Brazil. The Evandro Chagas Institute certified as positive the tests conducted on 16 people who presented preliminary results for the virus. Eight samples were from Bahia and eight from Rio Grande do Norte.

Brazilian Ministry of Health, Portal da Saúde

### SEPTEMBER 23, 2015

I lived in Natal until August 2015. I'd like to inform you that I caught the Zika virus in May. I was three months pregnant at the time, three months on the dot, my last period was on February 27. I was worried at the time and called my gynecologist to ask for some information or find out if there was a cure, because I was pregnant and really worried. I went back home to my country to finish out my pregnancy, and I'm still having MRIs and ultrasounds, because my baby suffered a serious encephalic injury and today they confirmed that his whole brain is irreversibly compromised. It was caused by a virus, but even now they don't know if it was Zika, simply because my gynecologist and other Brazilian doctors back then told me it was an unknown virus. But they said it would in no way influence the baby in my uterus. Next week, I'm going to check into one of the most important tropical disease treatment centers. If you'd like, I'll keep you informed, because I think that in situations like mine, where the life of defenseless beings is involved, public health needs to pay greater attention and care.

Email from Sofia Tezza, in Italy, to Dr Kleber Luz

## SEPTEMBER 24, 2015

The investigations into Zika were very complicated. It was very hard for us to convince the health authorities that there was a new virus; it wasn't easy. I'd like to know whether it was ever confirmed that your infection was caused by the virus.

Email from Dr Kleber Luz, in Natal, Brazil, to Sofia Tezza

## SEPTEMBER 24, 2015

Dear Dr Kleber, the gynecologist back then neither confirmed nor denied it, but he stated that it was a new virus and the symptoms were those of Zika, an unknown disease in my country. I studied it myself, because nothing has been published about it, but there's really no sure reference. But is this virus communicable? I caught it in May, my baby is compromised, but can I transmit it to my family? Thank you for your time.

Email from Sofia Tezza to Dr Kleber Luz

## NOVEMBER 11, 2015

The Minister of Health, by the legal powers vested in him under sections I and II, sole paragraph, art. 87 of the Constitution and, considering the changes in the epidemiological pattern of incidents of microcephaly in Pernambuco, with an observed increase in the number of cases and an unusual clinical pattern . . . hereby resolves to . . . declare a Public Health Emergency of National Concern.

Administrative ruling no. 1.813, Brazilian Ministry of Health

## NOVEMBER 17, 2015

I spoke with my two patients, and they were willing to help continue this research into the virus. We couldn't stand not having anything to tell our patients anymore. They wanted to know exactly what caused it. It was distressing not knowing what led to these cases.

Dr Adriana Melo, G1 online news service, Paraíba

## NOVEMBER 21, 2015

On November 17, 2015, Fiocruz [Oswaldo Cruz Foundation] reported that the Oswaldo Cruz Institute's Flavivirus Laboratory had completed diagnostic testing that detected the presence of the Zika virus genome in samples from two pregnant women from

Paraíba, whose ultrasound exams confirmed that their fetuses had microcephaly. Genetic material (RNA) from the virus was detected in samples of amniotic fluid using real-time RT-PCR. Although this is an important scientific finding as far as understanding Zika virus infection in humans, current data do not allow for the establishment of a causal relationship between Zika virus infection and microcephaly.

*Informe Epidemiológico* no. 01, 2015, Ministry of Health

## DECEMBER 1, 2015

Epidemiological Alert: Neurological syndrome, congenital malformations, and Zika virus infection. Implications for public health in the Americas.

Pan American Health Organization

## FEBRUARY 1, 2016

In assessing the level of threat, the 18 experts and advisers looked in particular at the strong association, in time and place, between infection with the Zika virus and a rise in detected cases of congenital malformations and neurological complications. The experts agreed that a causal relationship between Zika infection during pregnancy and microcephaly is strongly suspected, though not yet scientifically proven . . . . I am now declaring that the recent cluster of microcephaly cases and other neurological disorders reported in Brazil, following a similar cluster in French Polynesia in 2014, constitutes a Public Health Emergency of International Concern.

World Health Organization

## FEBRUARY 11, 2016

In mid-October 2015, a 25-year-old previously healthy European woman came to the Department of Perinatology at the University Medical Center in Ljubljana, Slovenia, because of assumed fetal anomalies. Since December 2013, she had lived and worked as a volunteer in Natal, the capital of Rio Grande do Norte state. She had become pregnant at the end of February 2015. During the 13th week of gestation, she had become ill with high fever, which was followed by severe musculoskeletal and retroocular pain and an itching, generalized maculopapular rash. Since there was a ZIKV epidemic in the community, infection with the virus was suspected, but no virologic diagnostic testing was performed. Ultrasonography that was performed at 14 and 20 weeks of gestation showed normal fetal growth and anatomy . . . . The clinical presentation raised suspicion of fetal viral infection. Because of severe brain disease and microcephaly, the fetus was given a poor prognosis for neonatal health. The mother requested that the pregnancy be terminated, and the procedure was subsequently approved by national and hospital ethics committees. Medical termination of the pregnancy was performed at 32 weeks of gestation . . . . This case shows severe fetal brain injury associated with ZIKV infection with vertical transmission.

Jernej Mlakar et al., *The New England Journal of Medicine*

## MARCH 17, 2016

How did your baby's story end?

Email from Dr Kleber Luz to Sofia Tezza

## APRIL 6, 2016

I never answered the Italian woman [when she wrote to me in 2015].
I was certain there was no chance it was Zika.

Interview with Dr Kleber Luz

## APRIL 7, 2016

Emergencies. Zika situation report. Zika virus, Microcephaly,
and Guillain-Barré syndrome . . . . Based on a growing body of
preliminary research, there is scientific consensus that Zika virus is
a cause of microcephaly and Guillain-Barré syndrome.

World Health Organization

## JUNE 8, 2016

My baby, Pietro, was getting quieter every day. I was in the
seventh month of my pregnancy, and nobody had anything certain
to say about the chances he would survive after birth or not. I went
to Slovenia. And in my eighth month, on October 13, 2015, Pietro
died. Labor was induced on October 15. I gave my baby to the
institute and months later they managed to find the virus's DNA.
Slovenia was the only place where I was treated like a human being,
and my baby too. They organized a celebration there, along with
other babies who flew off to heaven, because babies have to be
together.

Sofia Tezza, Italy

# Where the story unfolded in Brazil

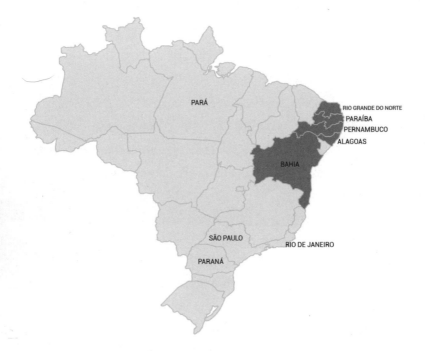

## Paraíba and Pernambuco

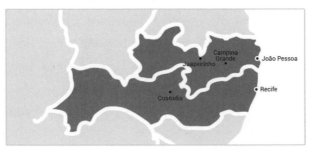

# TELLING THE STORY

This book follows Brazil's Zika epidemic as it unfolded in two somewhat overlapping chapters: the detection of a virus new to the country and the discovery that Zika can cause fetal microcephaly.[1] The account has been drawn directly from human experience: women's experiences with their own bodies and people's experiences within their families and communities, ranging from remote towns in rural Paraíba to the broader realm of Brazilian and world science. Within this framework, these pages tell how doctors and scientists in Brazil followed the trail of a new disease, interacted with their peers, and navigated the waters of science, government, and the press. Their stories are inextricably bound up with the stories of the women whose babies were struck by Zika before leaving the uterus, and they too feature prominently in this telling.

The narrative voice belongs to me, a Brazilian woman who made countless trips to Northeast Brazil to hear and record people's stories. I experienced this time with Zika in two ways, personally and professionally. While doing research for my documentary *Zika*,[2] I contracted the illness and suffered its textbook joint pain and skin rash. As someone who works with public health and bioethics, and above all as a woman listening to stories, I witnessed firsthand the anguish of pregnant women and caregivers of newborns as they faced a frightening unknown. As I traveled through the Northeast, I grew to understand that Zika, on one level, has become yet another health nuisance for people in the tropics, while on another, it now presents a dread peril for all women of reproductive age.

The setting is the Northeast, Brazil's poorest region, and the lead characters are Northeastern doctors, scientists, and ordinary women. For too many years, the Northeast was home to sugarcane plantations sustained by slavery. The states hit by Zika were also the site of the country's earliest universities and of train tracks laid by the British. The region produced Brazil's first abolitionists. Today, the Northeast can be thought of as divided between the coast and the *sertão* – the term for the parched rural areas that dominate the interior. When Zika struck, it was the inhabitants of the *sertão* who suffered most, far from the eyes of anyone enjoying a day at the beach.

Even more specifically, I followed people affected by the epidemic in five states within the Northeast, where its impact was harshest: Alagoas, Bahia, Paraíba, Pernambuco, and Rio Grande do Norte (see map on p. xx). On December 26, 2015, Paraíba led Brazil in the rate of reported cases of microcephaly, with 82.75 per 10,000 live births, while Pernambuco ranked a close second, with 80.38 per 10,000. Additionally, the first wave of Brazilian scholarship on the Zika epidemic and microcephaly came from physicians in Paraíba, Pernambuco, and Bahia.

The people of the *sertão* are known for their warmth and generosity and, to my good fortune in writing this book, they are consummate story tellers. While it was heartrending to see how the epidemic had devastated their forgotten, anonymous region, it was also enthralling to hear them weave their accounts, many extending interviews for hours, introducing me to their families, inviting me to join them for a dinner of cuscuz, showing me copies of text messages exchanged with other mothers or scientists, and sharing the details of scientific controversies. My Northeastern roots helped little; no one recognized mine as a regional accent, as time has stripped it of its Alagoan notes. If anything made a difference, it was the fact that I was a woman listening to stories of maternity, birth, or anguish over a sick child, to the Northeastern culture of motherhood being told and being heard.

There was a Brazilian, or perhaps Northeastern, touch to how science was done during these discoveries of Zika and its vertical transmission. Human warmth and solidarity often characterized interactions between the men and women who played leading roles. As science advanced, it walked hand in hand with religious beliefs. Dr Adriana Melo, an obstetrician from the state of Paraíba, and Géssica Eduardo dos Santos, the very first woman to donate amniotic fluid for Zika research, shared a sense of mission; they both responded to the epidemic by giving of themselves, though their belief systems differ: Dr Adriana is a Spiritist and Géssica is Catholic.

The Northeastern outlook was also visible in how mothers dealt with their situation. Some women said their children not only had Zika but *quebranto* as well. They explained it in these terms: "It's the evil eye . . . except when it attacks a child, you call it *quebranto*."[3] To break or mitigate the *quebranto* spell, the women said, you have to visit nine faith healers, known as *rezadeiras*. They also talked about the need for early stimulation, like exercises, activities, and other rehabilitation techniques to prevent or minimize delays in neuropsychomotor development. Among the many women I met were three from Juazeirinho, a city in Paraíba, whose children had been diagnosed with congenital Zika syndrome. One of them rebuffed the notion that a pesky mosquito had caused the disorder, insisting instead that she'd suffered a fright during pregnancy. She refused to take part in a medical research study, because she felt science could never explain what she already knew. Some of the researchers and doctors who I interviewed, especially in southern Brazil, scorned as scientific blasphemy the thinking of some Northeasterners. Others listened to these stories in solemn silence, and I wondered if they might not also be men and women who embrace traditional or folk modes of thought but had been regimented by the discourse of scientific neutrality.

In this story, where a mundane disease of the tropics proved to be a source of tremendous distress for women, the key protagonists were not physicians and scientists but these mothers-to-be. The outbreak of Zika itself was not a remarkable event. The disease has been known among humans in Africa and South Asia for over 50 years. And although Zika itself was a new word and a new disease in Brazil, *Aedes aegypti*, the vector that carries and transmits the virus, had been a member of the Brazilian household for over 40 years, ever since public health policy last eliminated the mosquito nationwide.[4] In part, this is why the baffling newcomer was first believed to be mild dengue. What was truly novel about Brazil's Zika epidemic was the associated microcephaly outbreak, a product of vertical transmission – that is, transmission of the illness by a pregnant woman to her fetus and the attendant possibility that the virus might adversely affect fetal development and cause permanent damage.

Dr Jernej Mlakar coordinated the team of Slovenian doctors who first detected the DNA of the Zika virus in a stillborn,[5] making use of the best technology available for researching human tissue. In Brazil, Dr Adriana Melo tested the hypothesis of vertical transmission by carefully studying the ailing bodies of women through the lens of her medical specialty and examining the amniotic fluid of two pregnant women.[6] There are clear-cut reasons why it was Dr Adriana and her team who substantiated the link between Zika and microcephaly in Brazil: she was trained to care for women and listen to the wisdom of mothers-to-be. "I just asked the question that my colleagues in Pernambuco hadn't. I looked at these pregnant women. But it was all right there in front of me," she stated, modestly implying that if it hadn't been her, it would have been some other researcher.

Science is urged on by controversy, and expressing doubt plays a valuable role in public discussion. In Brazil this is particularly true given generalized skepticism about national health surveillance data. While there have long been evident failings in the epidemiological reporting of newborns with microcephaly in Brazil, more to the point, there were no lengthy temporal series upon which comparisons could be based, because the disorder was new to Brazil; researchers would need to examine incoming data on a weekly basis, going back to the onset of the crisis. In point of fact, a more thoroughgoing analysis of the situation was only possible once Brazil's Ministry of Health had declared a Public Health Emergency of National Concern, on November 11, 2015.[7]

Some Brazilian researchers urged the use of consistent diagnostic criteria when investigating cases of suspected microcephaly.[8] Others wanted to believe that the numbers might prove in part an artifact of historical underreporting,[9] and they enlivened discussions in the press with basic lessons on how not to confuse a spurious correlation with causality[10] and how other countries were much more diligent about reporting microcephaly.[11] Neighboring countries challenged Brazil's numbers and the notion of a link between the Zika virus and microcephaly, alleging that it all boiled down to lax epidemiological surveillance; Brazil, they argued, had not properly monitored microcephaly in newborns and the Zika epidemic was merely the result of increased sensitivity to the problem.[12]

A report released by the Latin American Collaborative Study of Congenital Malformations (ECLAMC) described the spike in microcephaly cases in Northeast Brazil as "unprecedented" and listed among tentative causes for the surge the facts that (a) rumors about microcephaly had led to an active search for what were previously underreported cases; (b) reported cases included newborns with a normal head circumference because the cutoff for microcephaly was somewhat arbitrary; (c) errors were occurring in post-partum measurements; and (d) the cases were actually attributable to other causes.[13] While the method used to determine head circumference in Brazil is common practice worldwide – a measuring tape is wrapped around the newborn's head right in the delivery room – an epidemic indeed heightens people's sensitivity to a given phenomenon, and thus many cases of microcephaly might well have signaled previous overreporting.[14]

Skepticism about the numbers also reflected skepticism about the idea that Northeast Brazil can produce serious science. Not only were these Northeasterners mistrusted because of their geographic origins; many were also the target of suspicion because they were clinicians, professors, and healthcare providers lacking the usual scientific credentials listed in the bios published in high-impact international journals, which are often home to Nobel laureates.

And yet, since the Zika epidemic, the world has been hearing directly from this region, shaking Brazil's intellectual pecking order.

When I first took up this book project, I was inspired by classic works on the history of science, and I wanted to understand whether the events I was observing constituted a scientific revolution or whether this was merely a moment when an extraordinary event was reinvigorating the prevalent way of doing medical science – what Thomas Kuhn called *"normal science."*[15] I found no event that altered scientific thinking; rather, the pieces of the scientific puzzle were simply slipped into their proper place. Guillain-Barré syndrome (GBS) had been described decades earlier, so some of the neurological effects of the Zika virus were already known.[16] Zika is an arbovirus of the genus Flavivirus,[17] and there are other flaviviruses, like West Nile virus and Japanese encephalitis, that also affect the nervous system.[18] In public health terms, the initial challenge was to learn which of the flaviviruses was circulating in Brazil in the guise of mild dengue. Once Zika was discovered, the next steps followed quickly, and they were groundbreaking: the hypothesis was launched that the virus could not only lead to temporary paralysis in children and adults but also cross the placenta and irreversibly damage the fetus. But this hypothesis was grounded in what had already been predicted by the puzzle. There was no scientific revolution but rather a series of discoveries made within the bounds of everyday science.

If detection of the Zika virus in Brazil and the discovery of vertical transmission reflected good practice in normal science rather than a major scientific upheaval, there was still something momentous about the history of Zika in Brazil: there was a shift in the geography of legitimate science within the country's borders. The doctors who announced to the world the discovery of the new disease were from the Northeast, an area many Brazilians consider inferior within the national landscape. Southern Brazil, site of the top universities and research centers, finally had to pay heed to Northeastern scientists and physicians as they explained what they observed and discovered. This time, recognition for a major medical discovery made in Brazil went not to authorities in Rio de Janeiro or São Paulo, beneficiaries of the nation's most generous funding, but to authorities who touted their feats in the lilting accent of the Northeast. They were clinicians and practitioners of bedside medicine – where the focus is on the doctor–patient relationship – many of whom were unknown to the public at large or the academic community. It was these doctors' intimate contact with a tragedy that transformed them into scientists and projected them into the international spotlight as discoverers of a new ailment. Furthermore, the mothers of the babies with microcephaly were also poor Northeasterners, many of them farm workers, many black and brown, women whose faces and biographies are usually all but invisible in Brazil's socially stratified world.

In methodological terms, I conducted an ethnographic study. From February to June 2016, I spent stretches of time in Campina Grande, Paraíba, where I had daily contact with healthcare providers and women. I conducted 31 interviews and engaged in countless private conversations with doctors and scientists. In addition to interviewing these Northeasterners, I also observed and interacted with them; I sat in on appointments, spent time in waiting rooms, traveled to towns in the countryside. For many months now, I've been a member of two WhatsApp groups of mothers of children with microcephaly. There is only one topic in their daily exchanges of texts, audios, pictures, prayers, and chain letters: the special needs of these women's children, their pilgrimages to secure social assistance benefits, and the challenges they face with transportation and other logistical matters. In sharing their daily lives, I saw how the domestic science of caregiving advances alongside the official science of medicine.[19] Before medicine had figured it out, for example, many mothers suspected that their babies' constant crying was not just irritability but convulsions, and that their babies were not seeing or hearing like their age-mates.

My interviewees did not include the authors of the earliest publications on the Zika outbreak that took place in the Federated States of Micronesia, on Yap Island, in 2007.[20] Nor did I go back to primary sources from the early twentieth century, when GBS was first identified,[21] or from the 1940s, when the Zika virus was detected in Uganda.[22] My sources for these events were the academic articles and other peer-to-peer communications that form the official history of science. I did a review of the literature on PubMed[23] and also monitored 5,000 Brazilian and international media sources covering the period from October 2014 through June 2016, scouring thousands of articles on Zika, microcephaly, and congenital Zika syndrome. As a research strategy, following these reports allowed me both to track the public appearances and statements of the scientists and physicians interviewed in these pages and to confirm information on dates and places. Moreover, because the epidemic created a sense of urgency and because Brazilian doctors publish little in English-language journals, discoveries were first broadcast through the press and only later published by scientific periodicals.[24] I also attended dozens of academic seminars in Brazil and abroad.

Whenever we delve into unexplored terrain in examining an illness, it is helpful to rely on science's traditional problem-solving approaches, while still arming ourselves with a healthy dose of doubt. This was how I proceeded in my research. I monitored the mounting number of recent releases in the biomedical literature. Nothing was published in 2007, when the first Zika epidemic struck outside Africa – after all, communication between scientific peers moves more slowly than any public health emergency. Two articles came out in 2008, both on the outbreak on Yap Island. If journal articles can be considered a measure, the academic community's interest in the Zika virus then held steady for several years, until soaring in 2016: two articles were published in 2009; none in 2010; one in 2011; four in 2012; three in 2013; 23 in 2014; 41 in 2015; and 646 from January to June 2016.

This precipitous rise in the production of knowledge reflected the scientific community's reaction to the unfolding crisis. Certain Brazilians assumed a new status as often-cited authors in the discussion, like Dr Adriana Melo, mentioned earlier, until then not a scientist but a practicing clinician in Paraíba, or Dr Carlos Brito, from Pernambuco, previously known in Brazil as a dengue expert but, since October 2015, also a specialist on Zika who travels Latin America. Still, while Brazilian scientists were respectably represented in the pages of international journals in 2016, they accounted for no more than 8 percent of the hundreds of researchers who wrote about Zika. Furthermore, after Northeastern scientists announced their discoveries in the first round of scholarship, researchers in the country's large urban centers in the South started dominating articles authored by Brazilians.

This book was written almost in real time, during the second chapter of the epidemic. There was a pressing need to tell the story, yet its telling demanded delicacy even more than speed. I have documented records for almost all information presented here, but many of the facts and dates were recorded during interviews and, in a very few cases, there was no supporting documentation; given the frailty of human memory, this means there may be some inaccuracies. I asked interviewees to send me records of their conversations whenever possible, such as emails or text messages. In the few cases where these were not available, I still chose to share this material because I believe it is vital to register the memories of those who bear eye-witness to history. Lastly, these pages may contain some debatable versions of stories, since scientific discoveries do not take place in a vacuum; instead, they are part of a huge jigsaw puzzle being assembled by various players simultaneously. While the Brazilian researchers and doctors on this stage displayed tremendous camaraderie, the episodes and events were not without some resentments and disagreements. When faced with divergences between scientists, I sometimes had to choose between narrators or viewpoints.

While I was listening to these people, asking them questions, and mingling with them socially, I too was speaking out about the Zika epidemic. For anyone who believes that science is neutral, this book was contaminated from the outset, because I belong to a community of researchers, physicians, and scientists who have been involved with the epidemic in Brazil. I believe that the notion of neutrality has proven to be science's finest tool for boosting the tremendous authority wielded by scientists. I lay full claim to my own involvement, which was strategic to my efforts to wend my way through these mazes of people, institutions, and episodes.

I wish to leave clear that there were two levels to this engagement. On the one hand, the physicians and scientists who I interviewed were largely unaware of my activism and my own research. As far as many of them were concerned, my professional titles meant little; theirs was a world of mosquitoes in a laboratory or uteruses and new-borns in a delivery room. For the women, I was someone who had "come from Brasilia," the federal capital, to find out about their story, someone who listened attentively and patiently. At the same time, my Brazilian voice on the Zika epidemic and its women had an audience in arenas of research and activism abroad, and this facilitated my investigations in Brazil and my exchange with colleagues overseas.

In December 2015, the Pan American Health Organization invited me to join a work group assigned to draw up health recommendations on the reporting and surveillance of GBS and microcephaly.[25] This was my first participation in an international group as a specialist on the topic and my contribution was timid; I learned more than I shared. That said, while epidemiologists and specialists in children's health were expressing their concerns over how to measure a newborn's head circumference or what criteria should be used to make an early differential diagnosis of Zika, I insisted on the need to talk to women about reproductive health. The group completed its work in January 2016, and by that time it was clear that an unprecedented epidemic was laying siege to Brazil. On February 1, 2016, the World Health Organization (WHO) declared a Public Health Emergency of International Concern related to increased neurological disorders and fetal malformations associated with Zika, triggering a sensation of global threat because of the risk presented to pregnant women by the Zika virus.[26] That month, the group of activists and researchers that I coordinate announced that we would be filing suit to guarantee the rights of the women affected by the epidemic.[27] As of this writing, the case is still pending and will contribute to the third chapter of the history of the epidemic and its consequences for Brazilian women's reproductive health. In April 2016, I traveled to Washington DC to take part in a meeting of bioethics specialists convened by the Pan American Health Organization, where the document "*Zika ethics consultation:* ethics guidance on key issues raised by the outbreak" was drawn up.[28] I am pledged to confidentiality about the discussions that took place there, but the document itself speaks to my presence when it states:

> Taking into account the significant mental anguish about reproductive issues that women experienced during the Zika virus outbreak, along with the ethical duties to minimize harms and to allow for decisions to be made on the basis of the beliefs, values, situation, and concrete reality of each woman, the capacity to choose should include the full set of options including contraception and termination of pregnancy.[29]

My travels through the Northeast allowed me unique personal contact with doctors in the areas hit by Zika and with victims of the epidemic. Grounded in history as it was experienced and narrated, this is an eye-witness account from inside the epidemic itself. Today, in the aftermath of these events, I remain committed to further filling in gaps in my knowledge by listening hard and discovering what remains to be told about the struggles of the women of Northeast Brazil and their children in the era of Zika.

# POSITIVE FOR ZIKA

## WHERE IT ALL BEGAN

We Brazilians like to joke about our tragedies. Humor is a way of coping with the unbearable. Foreigners must find it curious when we say with a smirk, "We lost the World Cup in 2014 but we won Zika." This isn't exclusive to Brazilians; I'd dare say it's a Latin American way of exorcising disaster. The political climate in Brazil wasn't the most auspicious on the eve of the long-awaited soccer championship, held in 12 stadiums across the country from June 12 to July 13, 2014. Money was siphoned off into myriad pockets during the construction of sporting arenas and an anti-Cup movement bloomed across the country. Yet while many decried the soccer festival, there was a subtext of hope emblazoned across every team T-shirt and blasted through every noisy horn in the stadiums.

Despite the prevailing climate of under-confidence, Brazil's big dream was to secure the Cup right at home. Disappointment, however, came fast; the team only made it into the semi-finals and then had to settle for fourth place. Some even say Brazil's political crisis roared into its final phase following the country's disgraceful 7-1 loss to Germany. National pride suffered even more when arch-rival Argentina reached the finals. Much to the relief of the

Brazilian fans who refuse to root for their neighbors, Argentina lost to Germany in a hard-fought final game decided on penalty kicks.

There are strong competing hypotheses about how the Zika virus entered Brazil. It may have been via the FIFA World Cup. Some think it was during the Va'a World Sprint Championship, an outrigger canoe race that took place August 12–17, 2014 in Rio de Janeiro.[1] And there's a third hypothesis, which is that the virus arrived along with the FIFA Confederations Cup, held June 15–30, 2013, over two-and-a-half years before the official announcement that Zika had been detected in Brazil. This is a story with many versions. I offer them in these pages because they form the fabric of narratives embraced by serious researchers and physicians.

Zika originated in western Africa, later spreading to the rest of the continent and into Asia and producing different phylogenetic lineages;[2] three had been described as of June 2016: MR766 (isolated in Uganda in 1947), Nigerian, and Asian.[3] As part of the effort to determine which of these events actually introduced Zika, researchers sequenced the DNA of the strain circulating in Brazil, which proved to contain 99 percent Asian lineage, or genotype. Scientists do not know the identity of patient zero in Brazil – that is, the person who first carried Zika into the country – but given the fact that the Brazilian virus shares a common ancestor with the Asian strain, the conjecture became that Zika entered during either the FIFA Confederations Cup or the outrigger canoe championship, both of which brought athletes from French Polynesia, where an outbreak struck in late 2013 and continued into 2014.[4]

The group of scientists who identified the Brazilian strain defended the hypothesis that Zika arrived with the Confederations Cup, roughly in parallel with the outbreak on the other side of the world. They argued that the lag between the virus's entrance around June 2013 and its identification in 2015 could be attributed to the fact that Zika symptoms were at first confused with those of dengue or chikungunya; after all, as they saw it, "reliable differential diagnosis is possible only by using improved surveillance and laboratory diagnostics, which are now being implemented throughout the country."[5]

There is an interesting twist to the hypotheses about the arrival of the Zika virus, or ZIKV. As reported in the journal *Science*, "although the molecular clock dates are more consistent with the Confederations Cup tournament, that event ended before ZIKV cases were first reported in French Polynesia."[6] In other words, if Zika indeed entered Brazil during the Confederations Cup, this means the virus landed here before the outbreak had even been detected in French Polynesia, homeland of the alleged patient zero.

Dr Carlos Brito is a general practitioner and epidemiologist in Recife, capital of Pernambuco. His bedside experience has made him skeptical of the hypothesis that the virus accompanied the Confederations Cup into Brazil in 2013; instead, he believes it arrived in June 2014 via the World Cup. Why would the virus have landed, found an abundant supply of mosquitoes, and then spent a year resting before going on to sicken huge numbers of people? "This virus doesn't wait for the next Cup or the next game. It's shown us that. It makes its move in the first half; it doesn't wait for overtime," Dr Brito told me, explaining what he believes laboratory scientists miss when it comes to the logic of diseases. In early 2015, Dr Brito began treating swarms of people with skin rashes and body aches that apparently had no relation to dengue or chikungunya, and he built his hypotheses on this contact with the people actually stricken by the disease.

The belief that a diagnosis is only reliable if proven by laboratory tests was one of the points of controversy surrounding the epidemic and it has a direct bearing on how science is done and medicine practiced. An epidemic breeds agreements and disagreements between healthcare providers and laboratory scientists; bedside physicians murmur their hypotheses into the ears of scientists, who hunt for evidence to prove or refute the concerns of these clinicians. For scientists in their lab coats laboring over microscopes, truths must be proved through repeated tests of their own, later replicated by other researchers. For a practicing physician, there are other ways of evincing scientific truths in medicine, and clinical diagnosis based on a personal encounter with the patient is considered just as important as laboratory evidence. This is what is known as an epidemiological link: when a case satisfies the clinical definition for a certain ailment and has a direct link to a laboratory-confirmed case of the same ailment.

It is from the perspective of these conflicting approaches to medicine that Dr Brito disputes the hypothesis that Zika came to Brazil via the Confederations Cup in 2013, a year and a half before people started falling ill. "This argument reflects a lack of clinical experience. The clinical characteristics of these illnesses [dengue, chikungunya, and Zika] in epidemic form are completely different. The fact is that when [Zika] showed up in Brazil for the first time, in 2015, we immediately recognized that it wasn't dengue or chikungunya and for months we insisted on that," the physician says. He rejects the notion that the phylogenetic lineage of the virus sets the historical timeframe of its arrival in Brazil, just as he rejects the idea that the arbovirus remained latent and then, in the space of a few months, crossed borders to become a global threat.

The term *"arthropod-borne viruses"* was introduced in 1942 to describe viruses transmitted by arthropods, two examples of which are insects and arachnids. The shortened form *"arboviruses"* was adopted in 1963.[7] The Centers for Disease Control and Prevention (CDC) has recorded the existence of over 500 arboviruses worldwide.[8] The only continent free of endemic arboviruses is Antarctica.[9] They are more prevalent in the tropics, where climate and environment favor their dissemination.[10]

The Zika virus is an arbovirus of the genus Flavivirus, which encompasses more than 50 other species, including dengue, yellow fever, St Louis encephalitis, and West Nile virus.[11] It is no surprise that the Amazon rainforest is one of the largest arbovirus reservoirs on the planet; over 200 types circulate in Brazil and almost all of them were first detected in the Amazon. Only a little over 30 have been recognized as causing sickness in humans.[12]

The Zika virus was first isolated from a sentinel rhesus monkey in 1947 as part of a study on yellow fever.[13] It was isolated from humans in 1952 in Uganda and since then it has been found in over 76 countries and territories; in 59 of these, the first outbreak occurred after 2015.[14] Named after the forest in Uganda where it was first detected, Zika means "overgrown" in the Luganda language, which belongs to the Bantu family.[15] For those who like precise figures, the medical literature reports only 13 or 14 cases of human sickness from the first record of Zika in humans to the 2007 Yap Island outbreak.[16] This all changed in the wake of Yap, which was followed by the 2013 outbreak in French Polynesia and the one in Brazil in 2015.

In 2007, Zika triggered epidemics both in Gabon, where the vector was the *Aedes albopictus* mosquito, and on Yap Island.[17]

Estimates suggest that about 5,000 of the island's 7,391 inhabitants were infected.[18] The disease was first thought to be dengue, but because two prior dengue outbreaks had left physicians trained in diagnosing this illness, they realized the symptoms they were seeing weren't a perfect fit.[19] In June, doctors there sent the CDC 71 blood samples from individuals in the acute phase of the illness; Zika was detected in 10.[20] During the large outbreak in French Polynesia in 2013, an estimated 28,000 people were infected, or 11.5 percent of the population.[21] French Polynesia brought something unprecedented: it was reported that Zika patients also developed GBS.[22]

Very little was known about Zika prior to the epidemic in Brazil. Following this outbreak, research about Yap Island and French Polynesia was supplemented by retrospective analyses, with scientists returning to previously collected data, blood samples, and medical reports in order to describe what had happened, test hypotheses about the neurological changes noted in adults, like GBS, and look for cases of fetal microcephaly.[23]

My point in relating these competing hypotheses about the arrival of Zika in Brazil is to highlight scientific interest in the origin of the disease. But these stories should be repeated with caution because the search for a patient zero is always risky,[24] as the world has seen with HIV and Ebola in Africa. Moreover, there is a danger of assigning stigma to individuals or blaming them for events that are actually collective in nature. In fact, these accounts may be more pertinent to the quest for mythical origins than to the practice of serious science.

There would have been no epidemic like the one in Brazil had the land not been hospitable to the explosive spread of the disease thanks to its mosquito populations, poor sanitation, and feeble public health policies for addressing new diseases. The mosquito vector had been waiting more than 40 years for a new virus to come along so it could transmit sickness to virgin populations. Zika would not have assumed tragic dimensions in Brazil nor would chikungunya have spread across the country in the second half of 2014 if the mosquito were not found in every last corner of the country.[25]

Brazil had managed to eliminate the *Aedes aegypti* mosquito in the 1950s.[26] The key control method was the same used today: destroying the vector and ensuring that the country's borders were free of the insect. But the pesky mosquito returned. In 1973, it was successfully eliminated again, for a two-time win. By 1976, however, it was back, never to leave. Experts blame this on failings in epidemiological surveillance and on booming urbanization; perhaps global warming plays a role as well.[27] Whatever the explanation, the reality is this: two victories for public health were followed by the mosquito's triumphant return over 40 years ago. This is why talking about a patient zero in the case of Zika in Brazil is much less relevant than talking about the vector's persistence.

## DECIPHERING AN ALLERGY EPIDEMIC

Chikungunya was expected in Brazil. They say it slipped in through more than one door, in September 2014: Oiapoque, in the state of Amapá, and Feira de Santana, Bahia, a hub of trade and travel between southern Brazil and the North and Northeast. These two entrances are relevant because Brazil has two lineages of the chikungunya virus, or CHIKV, the shorthand term used by scientists and physicians; the Asian genotype entered via Oiapoque while the African came in through Feira de Santana.[28]

Dr Kleber Luz is a practicing pediatrician, epidemiologist, and professor at the Federal University of Rio Grande do Norte. He is one of those rare professors and researchers who has never forgotten that close contact with patients is the best way to practice medicine. During the Zika epidemic in Brazil, other doctors in the region often turned to him with questions about clinical symptoms and diagnoses. His qualifications recently earned him an invitation to spend a semester as consultant to the Pan American Health Organization in Washington, DC. He was also one of the Brazilians trained to diagnose chikungunya in Paraguay in 2012 and in Martinique in 2014. The appearance of the virus in the Caribbean had foreshadowed its imminent arrival in Brazil.

At the outset of the epidemic, news reports on chikungunya fever pointed to the need to differentiate its symptoms from those of dengue, a focus that would be repeated during the Zika epidemic. G1, a major online news service in Brazil, titled one report "Signs of chikungunya fever resemble those of dengue; get to know the disease."[29] On September 16, 2014, the Ministry of Health issued its first alert regarding autochthonous transmission: chikungunya had been passed on inside the country.

Dr Kleber has a research partner in Dr Carlos Brito, from Pernambuco. Both men knew that chikungunya would spread quickly through the Northeast, with a stampede of patients seeking medical attention. The illness causes severe muscle aches, persistent malaise, and often times high fever. Bridging clinical practice and epidemiology, a WhatsApp group called "CHIKV, the mission" was created to keep a broad network of doctors informed. According to Dr Brito, the group was the brainchild of Rodrigo Said, a staff member at Pernambuco's state health surveillance agency and coordinator of the first medical inspection team to visit Feira de Santana.

The group adopted the term "mission" because of the weight of the tasks looming before its members. Not only would they gather material and make diagnoses; they would likewise draft a chikungunya protocol for the Ministry of Health. The term was also an allusion to the 1986 movie *The Mission*, an allegorical depiction of Jesuit missionary priests in seventeenth-century Argentina and Paraguay.[30] We might say that the first doctors who ventured into Brazil's interior to study the illness merged professional and personal concerns; they were imbued with the spirit of science but also with a sense of spiritual mission, perhaps drawing inspiration from the religious symbolism of salvation. Since the birth of "CHIKV, the mission" in October 2014, Dr Brito has been one of the group's most energetic forces. He and Dr Kleber could never have foreseen how much of the history of the Zika virus would be threaded through the group's messages.[31]

Observing with trained eyes the symptoms of what was assumed to be chikungunya, clinicians in the Northeast began to sense that something was wrong. Many patients had low-grade fevers and rashes that left them itching all over, symptoms that frequently vanished in a few days. Dr Celso Tavares is a friend of Dr Kleber's. His name is not to be found in news reports on CHIKV or ZIKV in Brazil. As a clinician specializing in infectious diseases in Alagoas, he crisscrosses the state visiting the sick. It was during a trip to Mata Grande, a forgotten town on the border with Pernambuco, that he began suspecting that a new disease might be circulating. "The first thing that bugged me was that the patients didn't have high fevers," he wrote in a letter to Dr Kleber. People were describing their malaise as an "awful allergy," and drugstore shelves had been cleared of antihistamines. Dr Celso finds it no wonder that pharmacies serve as surrogate clinics in the Northeast. "Public healthcare clinics don't offer much of anything other than what you find at a drugstore," he explained.

Dr Celso says he became "obsessed" as he made the rounds of Mata Grande. He recalled Brazilian geographer Milton Santos and his words about the world having grown smaller with the circulation of so many new diseases. "It's as if the world were now within everyone's grasp," Santos wrote.[32] Dr Celso was convinced these people were not suffering from an allergy, because multiple cases would appear in a single family. The first patient he remembers was a woman who described her symptoms with these words: "A whole bunch of ants biting me. Just like an ant bite. And then it goes away in a while and the ant shows up somewhere else." Another patient said there was "something running up and down [her] calf, ripping it." While pondering the disease and the words of Milton Santos, Dr Celso made more trips deep into Alagoas. "The 'awful allergy' was spreading across towns in the interior," he told me. In December 2014, he called Dr Kleber.

The two men initiated a steady stream of correspondence, exchanging images and information about their patients' clinical signs and complaints. To one of his text messages, Dr Celso attached photographs of the skin rashes presented by a number of patients. This rash – or exanthema, in medical terms – was the key sign that something other than a typical virus was attacking the body. The photos feature shots of legs, soles of feet, cheeks – a collection of body parts that would hopefully help in deciphering the new disease. As Dr Kleber scrolled quickly through the images during one of our conversations, it brought to mind the wax models of body parts known as ex-votos that the devout sometimes place on altars, praying for a miracle. Dr Celso's pictures offered proof that the virus was present in the body of patients complaining of pain and itchiness. The two roaming physicians from Northeast Brazil were separated from each other by more than 500 kilometers, but technology linked them as if they worked in adjacent offices.

In some of the photos, the rashes seemed sparse and localized; in others, a sandpaper mantle of tiny bumps covered the body from palms of hands to soles of feet. People complained that they itched like crazy. Very often their eyes were red and streaked, a condition called conjunctivitis. In my mind, I tried to make up stories to go along with the images of these ex-votos, but the most I could figure out was if the parts belonged to a man or a woman or if the wrinkles or taut skin suggested someone younger or older.

Dr Kleber says that "tracking down diseases" is just part of his nature. He too was observing the growth of an unknown viral illness. This was around Natal, the state capital, and especially in Parnamirim, near the city's airport. He repeatedly asked his friend in Alagoas for more details and Dr Celso was always eager to reply. One time Dr Celso wrote:

When I got to Mata Grande, I spoke with two patients in the hospital and then with those at the walk-in clinic – with the ones who were sick, the convalescing, the cured. I want to stress that these data haven't been processed because my computer caught a nasty bug and I have no way of seeing the blood counts and other test results. I need your help. The disease has been raging since December 1, at least. It doesn't always start with a fever but with numbness and tearing, burning pain.

Dr Kleber was to make Dr Celso his principle sounding board when he later began suspecting that the viral illness was not an allergy and that it had a specific name in the arbovirus catalogue: Zika. ZIKV can transmit the disease many ways, but transmission via a mosquito vector is the most common. In the case of Brazil's threefold epidemic, dengue, chikungunya, and Zika have a vector in common, *Aedes aegypti*, a dark-colored mosquito with white markings on its legs that looks much like a tiny winged zebra. Every town visited by Dr Celso and Dr Kleber was infested with *Aedes aegypti*.

A variety of other mosquitoes can transmit ZIKV as well, including *Aedes polynesiensis*, *Aedes albopictus*, and *Aedes hensilli*, but those of the *Culicidae* family and specifically the genus *Aedes* are the most common transmitters. Of all mosquitoes, *Aedes aegypti* is the most efficient at transmitting Zika in a given location and time, for various reasons: (a) it feeds off human blood; (b) it can bite a number of people during a single meal, flitting inconspicuously from one victim to another; (c) its bite goes almost unnoticed; (d) human dwellings are its habitat; and (e) it feeds only in the daytime.[33] Less scientifically speaking, *Aedes aegypti* is just another member of the Brazilian family: its bite doesn't really bother anyone, it likes to take its meals with the rest of the folks, and it enjoys sharing a bedroom with company.

Dr Kleber began to seriously entertain the possibility that Brazil had a new arbovirus making the rounds. He noted marked similarities between the symptoms in patients from Parnamirim and the symptoms Dr Celso was reporting in the interior of Alagoas. The conjunctivitis, low-grade fever or no fever at all, and the speed with which the illness vanished were typical of neither dengue nor chikungunya. Dr Kleber showed me an email from Dr Celso, sounding like he'd recited the same story time and again. He told me to pay close attention to the time and date on the message: 14:05 pm, February 4, 2015. "Kleber," it read, "almost all municipalities are disregarding *Aedes* control, and in all of them surveillance is poor, as is health care, which makes early, proper diagnosis challenging." Dr Kleber replied: "There are a few flaviviruses and no sign of CHIKV, according to the Evandro Chagas Institute!"

Located in Belém, Pará, the Evandro Chagas Institute is a world-class center in the field of tropical medicine and a leading Brazilian laboratory in arboviruses. Today it is also the country's sentinel agency for Zika. The institute is named in honor of Evandro Chagas, a mid-twentieth-century researcher of leishmaniasis who died in a plane crash at an early age; he was the son of Carlos Chagas, another big name in the study of tropical diseases. The institute is part of the Oswaldo Cruz Foundation (known by its Portuguese acronym Fiocruz), Brazil's massive, government-owned public health research institution, with branches and agencies spread across the country. As one of the Ministry of Health's reference laboratories, the Evandro Chagas Institute is responsible for analyzing tropical diseases, both known and new, and so physicians had been sending blood samples to the laboratory in hopes of identifying the culprit behind the illness.[34] Many, like Dr Kleber, were eager for the institute to ratify their hypotheses and were growing frustrated because results never turned up anything but dengue. At the same time, the laboratory claimed that samples were being improperly handled by those collecting them.

Dr Celso sent his friend further descriptions of what he was observing on his visits:

> There was the allergy hypothesis in the beginning. What a run on antihistamines and steroids! There's frequent nausea but it's not intense; I haven't heard reports of vomiting; haven't seen hemorrhaging; haven't observed urinary, digestive, or respiratory involvement. . . . Other diseases are circulating there right now. Obviously, I don't think it's tied to water, or very contagious, or related to pesticides. I await your reply.

And he sent more photos to his friend, the disease hunter.

Dr Celso's rejection of the idea that there was any link to pesticides came months before rumors that pesticides or vaccines were causing a surge in microcephaly, a story that started circulating on social media in December 2015, during the second chapter of the history of ZIKV in Brazil.[35] Neither doctor thought twice about either possibility. They knew they were watching the vector *Aedes aegypti* on the move again, the same one that hadn't budged from Brazil in 40 years. The challenge was to discover which virus could cause symptoms resembling an allergy or mild dengue. At that moment in time, Zika was irrelevant as an epidemic threat.

Dr Kleber sought advice in the pages of an old green book on his shelves, *Manson's Tropical Diseases*, a classic manual of tropical medicine. Today's generations turn to the book for guidance when facing some pressing issue, but few know anything about the story of its author. Sir Patrick Manson, a nineteenth-century Scottish physician, was one of the founders of tropical medicine, a vast field that includes diseases transmitted by mosquitoes, like dengue, chikungunya, and Zika. Dr Kleber scoured the chapter on arbovirus infections, but there were so many that Zika got lost in the middle. In his edition, the few lines devoted to ZIKV began: "There are a large number of other arthropod viruses that only rarely cause human infection or where their role in human disease is uncertain."[36]

Doctors had been sending blood samples to laboratories since January 2015, but results kept coming back negative. Dengue was found in a few specimens but Dr Celso and Dr Kleber knew the symptoms didn't match up. Some of their academic colleagues insisted that they were dealing with mild dengue. Dr Kleber decided to revive the spirit of mission in the CHIKV group. He took a large team of students with him to Currais Novos, a town in Rio Grande do Norte on the border with Paraíba, where huge numbers were reported to be ailing from the unknown "allergy."

To avert potential criticism about sampling techniques, Dr Kleber made sure his team included researchers who were skilled in drawing blood. His critics questioned how the samples were handled because they had expected CHIKV to be found, not because they thought a new virus would be detected – much less ZIKV. Over 500 samples were collected, many of which were sent to the Evandro Chagas Institute. In the end, around 20 percent tested positive for dengue. The rest remained unexplained, but public health officials felt this evidence was "enough to say it was dengue," as Dr Kleber told me, somewhat disappointed by this apparent waste of time.

Dr Kleber was convinced that if it were dengue, people would be hospitalized or even dying. "We started to rethink chikungunya. It had to be a disease involving rash and itchiness, one that compromised the joints and was transmitted by *Aedes*." Armed with this information, he went back to Manson's green book, this time studying a table on mosquitoes and the arboviruses that transmit them. The table was divided into columns labeled virus, geographic distribution, transmission, and symptoms. ZIKV was on the list and the symptoms fit what Dr Kleber had observed in Currais Novos and as described by Dr Celso: skin rashes and joint pain. And once again, there was *Aedes*. Reading this set of symptoms, Dr Kleber re-interpreted the clues: "In my mind, it just had to be Zika." He claims that in more than one conference call with the Ministry of Health, he announced his hypothesis that they were encountering Zika but his observations went unheeded. This was during February and March 2015.

Unhappy with the Evandro Chagas Institute's inconclusive findings, Dr Kleber contacted Dr Cláudia Duarte dos Santos at a branch of Fiocruz's Oswaldo Cruz Institute located in Paraná, southern Brazil. Dr Cláudia is one of Brazil's most experienced researchers of viral diseases. She is a laboratory scientist trained not to examine a patient's body but the tiny parts of it that carry disease. The contact between her and Dr Kleber represented a meeting of the science of evidence with the science of determination, where the sensitive eye of a family doctor from the Northeast prompted a laboratory scientist in her white coat to probe the possibility of a new disease in Brazil. The blood samples from Currais Novos could have contained any virus, but she received them with a clinical diagnosis: "It's Zika. Find Zika," Dr Kleber told her.

While Dr Cláudia began performing real-time RT-PCR analyses to look for a variety of viruses in the blood samples, using generic rather than ZIKV-specific primers,[37] Dr Kleber continued exchanging messages about his Zika hypothesis. He went back to texting with his friend Dr Celso. On March 12, 2015, he wrote: "Hey fellow, any conclusions about your folks with exanthema?" To which Dr Celso replied, "My friend, I'm trying to figure out what the devil is going on. There's a new, unspecified flavivirus hanging around, but it doesn't fit the description of a Mayaro." Mayaro was one of the flaviviruses listed in Manson's book. On March 13, Dr Kleber prodded him: "Look at the description of the Zika virus. I think that's it."

By then, Dr Kleber was quite confident of his diagnosis. On the morning of March 13, he had gathered a group of professors and students for a class at the Federal University of Rio Grande do Norte School of Medicine and had asked each of them to test a diagnostic hypothesis about the circulating flavivirus. Using eight slides, he defended the thesis that it was Zika. Dr Kleber's computer saved the last change to his teaching plan for the class: 9:11 am, March 13, 2015. The class was held at 10:00 am, and his exchange with Dr Celso took place that afternoon. Dr Kleber had no more doubts. He only needed proof from another branch of science to back him up.

For his part, Dr Celso wrote to his friend Dr Pedro Fernando da Costa Vasconcelos, director of the Evandro Chagas Institute, reiterating his request for further investigation of the blood samples from Currais Novos: "Pedro, is Zika included in your battery? The situation is still the same here." Vasconcelos replied the same day, March 25, 2015, but without making a firm commitment: "No. But we could arrange primers for molecular detection." Primers are partial strings of DNA that are used in RT-PCR; each primer is designed to detect a specific virus or set of viruses. Dr Celso knew that laboratory investigations into any suspected disease must be guided by clinical information, which is why he pushed the Evandro Chagas Institute to move beyond their first generic results. He paraphrased the institute's reports to me: "'Dengue', and there in the corner, 'unspecified flavivirus'." The problem, however, is that dengue virus reacts to the generic tests, so if someone had been infected by the illness in the past, their blood would test positive for it, thus yielding many inconclusive results. Dengue was camouflaging Zika in the non-specific search for a flavivirus.

Within the "CHIKV, the mission" group, Dr Brito was forwarding Dr Kleber clinical descriptions similar to what Dr Celso was reporting in rural Alagoas.

Kleber, here in Recife we have an outbreak characterized by little or no fever, rash, and joint pain, with edema of the hands and ankles, mild in intensity but completely different from the intensity of chikungunya. . . . Healthcare providers . . . believe that another virus (ex.: parvovirus) should be investigated.

This clinical report – which could have been an updated version of the ZIKV section in Manson's manual – was accompanied by the image of a woman's extremely swollen fingers and palms. Dr Kleber's typically laconic reply left no room for doubt: "This must be the Zika virus. Look. Everybody here is sick. . . . It's got to be Zika." This exchange of messages took place on March 27, 2015.

Back at the Fiocruz laboratory in southern Brazil, Dr Cláudia was busy scrutinizing Dr Kleber's samples for the virus's genome, when, on April 29, 2015, the stunning announcement came that a husband and wife team of researchers, Dr Gúbio Soares Campos and Dr Silvia Sardi, had detected the Zika virus in blood samples from patients in Camaçari, Bahia. Dr Cláudia shifted from generic testing to perform tests specific to the DNA of the Zika virus; one week later, she detected ZIKV in eight of the fourteen samples from Currais Novos. On May 14, she announced her own findings, two weeks after the researchers in Bahia had gone to the press with theirs.

When Dr Cláudia and Dr Kleber had learned of the other scientists' feat, she had thoughtfully written to her colleague in northern Brazil: "I am so very sorry we failed. But we used the generic flavi primers and none of the samples you sent came out positive. . . . You were really very skilled in your diagnosis."[38] Indeed, Dr Kleber had been wiser than laboratory science, in a show of healthcare practice outpacing the test tube. Yet it was the couple in Bahia who took the national stage as the discoverers of Zika in Brazil.

When I spoke with Dr Cláudia, I insisted on knowing precisely who should get the credit for discovering the Zika virus in Brazil. She bristled at my question. With a mixture of pride and magnanimity, she said she didn't know who had actually been the first to identify it, her team in Paraná or the one in Bahia, but it didn't really matter much; what was uncontestable was that the paper that she, Dr Kleber, and other researchers went on to write was the first on the detection of ZIKV in Brazil to be published in a journal of international standing.[39] Still, in the course of our conversation, her feeling of injustice got the better of her and she eventually declared: "If you ask me who discovered the Zika virus in Brazil, I'll tell you: Kleber Luz."

Dr Cláudia had multiple reasons for taking umbrage when I pushed to know who had done what and when. Our depiction of the history of science and medicine tends to be misguided; we like to think in terms of lone, autonomous discoverers or reclusive geniuses. But as we have seen, that is not how this history is written.

## A MYSTERIOUS ILLNESS STRIKES BAHIA

While physicians like Dr Kleber, Dr Brito, and Dr Celso were busy decoding the outbreak of a new disease in Alagoas, Paraíba, Pernambuco, and Rio Grande do Norte Brazil, Bahia was likewise at the mercy of Zika – and likewise unaware of it. There too puzzled physicians had been trying to crack the case.

Dr Antônio Bandeira is a practicing physician who specializes in infectious diseases; he also teaches at a private college. He works in the city of Camaçari, some 50 kilometers north of Salvador, capital of Bahia. In January 2015, he started treating hordes of people stricken by what was variously described as Camaçari disease, Camaçari syndrome, or simply "a mysterious illness."[40] The town lies adjacent to a colossal chemical and petrochemical park, and the lay public surmised that the ailment was caused by pollution. Nobody talked about allergies, as they did in Dr Celso's corner of the Northeast, but about water contamination. The local health department explored the idea that they might be dealing with a parvovirus, a class of viruses transmitted by animals like dogs and pigs. Entire families had crowded Dr Antônio's office presenting symptoms similar to those of dengue or chikungunya, but their rashes were not typical of either. Instead, they presented "a lot of isolated spots."

In the late afternoon of March 26, 2015, Dr Antônio drove slowly through Salvador in the midst of a tropical downpour. Traffic had ground to a halt. His precious cargo was nestled in a bed of ice inside a small yellow Styrofoam cooler: 24 test tubes full of blood drawn from patients who had the mysterious illness. The samples had been collected three days earlier, and the local press had already reported that research had begun.[41] Dr Antônio had recruited the assistance of Dr Gúbio Soares Campos, a research colleague of his, for help investigating the disease. But the rain was keeping him from reaching Salvador. They agreed to meet at the airport. Dr Antônio admits he hadn't thought of Zika when he handed his colleague the cooler that housed the baffling illness. "At that point, I told him to follow this thought: it was a disease with a vector; it might be a mosquito or a tic. Some arbovirus." He gave Dr Gúbio the tubes of blood, along with a pen drive on which he had stored more than 300 photos of the ill – ex-voto body parts from Paraíba now finding echo in Bahia.

Dr Gúbio is a quiet man and a rather timid story-teller, unlike his talkative friend. He went on alone with the cooler, taking it to his tiny laboratory. With a floor space of just over 100 square meters, the facility is almost too small to hold all of its equipment plus the personnel who circulate there every day. And while it may be the finest virology laboratory at the Federal University of Bahia, it looks like a makeshift garage compared to its counterparts in southern Brazil. Nonetheless, with three PCR instruments, one real-time PCR system, and various freezers, it was equipped to detect the Zika virus. Dr Gúbio's lab partner, Dr Silvia, is also his partner at home. The couple met when he was doing his PhD in Buenos Aires. He holds a degree in pharmacy and she, in veterinary science, but both have made their careers as virologists. The couple decided to relocate to Bahia when she was expecting their first child and the economic crisis in Argentina was not auguring well for anyone pursuing a research career. After settling in Salvador, the couple established the laboratory.

Dr Silvia speaks fluent Portuguese, with a slight Buenos Aires accent over a slow Bahian drawl. She seems to be the one in charge, if not at home at least in the lab. Dr Gúbio, as the laboratory's unofficial public relations man, forges relationships with the few university physicians who are truly interested in research, and Dr Antônio ranked high among these. The couple began dedicating themselves to the mysterious illness and its ailing victims. This was how the cooler full of blood had ended up in the laboratory, carried by Dr. Gúbio. Dr Silvia was waiting for him, ready to embark on a new cycle of living and thinking together.

The husband and wife team started by reviewing the scientific literature. Dr Gúbio sat alone at the computer, reading recent publications on flaviviruses. Beside him was his copy of *Fields Virology*, a manual he calls the "virology bible."[42] ZIKV earns no more than 15 lines in the book, offering the same brief history as always: Uganda, discovery of the virus in rhesus monkeys, the role of vectors. Dr Silvia turned her attention to the matter of scientific instruments and the selection of primers. For 35 days, they poured themselves into their research. Their first discovery came partway through. "There are no samples with dengue. Nobody has dengue," Dr Gúbio texted Dr Antônio. He next confirmed the absence of the Mayaro, St Louis, and West Nile viruses.[43]

A laboratory scientist soon learns that when a test fails to confirm a hypothesis, it's time to move on to the next question. Science is not propelled by findings alone but by refuted premises, and the researchers knew that casting aside a string of hypotheses might simply mean they were edging closer to a discovery. Not finding dengue in the blood was the first result. The second, on April 22, was detecting CHIKV in three samples from the set of 24. This was breaking news, since no one realized Camaçari had been experiencing an outbreak of chikungunya since March 2015.

Dr Antônio wanted them to do more research. "Let's keep looking because there's more going on here," he said. He knew the legions of sick people in Camaçari did not have chikungunya and that CHIKV was merely an interloper along the path to a more important discovery. Dr Gúbio and Dr Silvia share similar recollections of these days of intense research. They spent more time at the lab than at home.

Dr Antônio left for a conference on infectious diseases in Denmark, from April 25 to 28, 2015.[44] He was still in Copenhagen when he received a text message from Dr Gúbio with an image of the test results: "I've analyzed six samples for the Zika virus, three from Camaçari and three from Aliança. I don't know everyone's symptoms. Only one sample from Camaçari tested positive for the Zika virus, and the symptoms in the literature match up. I'm going to start analyzing more samples tomorrow. I'm certain the outbreak is Zika."[45] It was 8:44 pm on April 28, 2015. Dr Antônio replied instants later: "Wow, incredible! I return to Brazil today."

Dr Antônio couldn't contain himself. He had been about to board his plane in Copenhagen when the message came in from Dr Gúbio. Before any official announcement had been made in Brazil, Dr Antônio shared the news with the foreign scientists around him: "'The mysterious illness is the Zika virus.' Everyone looked at me as if I were talking about a creature from another planet." Crowding around him in the departure lounge, his colleagues pestered him for more information: "What's that?" "What's Zika?" Dr Antônio had no inkling how many times he would answer that question going forward – much less how many times he, Dr Gúbio, and Dr Silvia would have to explain how three unknown scientists from Bahia had made a scientific discovery of worldwide importance.

Dr Silvia remembers the moment they told Dr Antônio the news: "He was on the other side of the planet and the first to know besides us." But she wasn't right there in the lab either. "Obviously, since we're a couple, I'm always the one who leaves first, to take care of our home and our son," she explained in the gentle voice of someone who divides herself between two worlds because that is what she wants and how she believes things should be. Although, right then, what she wanted to do was spend the whole night at the lab.

Both of them were back at it early the next morning, going through all the samples. Dr Gúbio had slept restlessly. He was completely confident of his message to his colleague – it was an outbreak of Zika. The couple did further testing and as Dr Antônio disembarked in Salvador, he read on his phone: "I detected Zika in three more samples." Then another message came in: "I detected Zika in another three samples." In the end, eight samples tested positive for ZIKV, but one of them was poorly identified and could not be used in reports or publications. All told, the Zika virus had been detected in seven people from Camaçari, Bahia. The mysterious illness had acquired an old name, and a frightening one.

Dr Gúbio announced their discovery to the press on April 29, 2015. "Virus discovered behind mysterious illness in Salvador and Metropolitan Region"[46] read one headline. Next he called Wanderson de Oliveira, then general coordinator of Surveillance and Response to Public Health Emergencies at the Ministry of Health. According to Dr Gúbio, a lengthy conversation ensued by speaker phone, with Dr Silvia and him on one end and Oliveira on the other, along with Dr Claudio Maierovich, then director of the ministry's Department of Communicable Disease Surveillance. As to why they were so quick to contact the press, Dr Gúbio says: "We decided to benefit the public more, rather than immediately writing a scientific paper and publishing it."

The skepticism began. The day after the discovery was announced, Dr Gúbio found himself juggling questions from reporters one moment and requests for information from fellow researchers the next. This included videoconference calls where he detailed the techniques his team had used to arrive at their findings. Dr Gúbio and Dr Silvia had used two primers to detect ZIKV, the first obtained from Oumar Faye, of the Pasteur Institute in Dakar, Senegal, and the second from Dr Michelle Balm, of National University Hospital in Singapore.[47] During a later phase of the epidemic, in January 2016 – by which time microcephaly had already been detected – Faye visited Brazil under a cooperation agreement between the University of São Paulo and scientists who had experience with Ebola and Zika in Africa.[48] The participation of the Senegalese team, even after the epidemic itself, stands as evidence that Dr Gúbio and Dr Silvia navigate trustworthy scientific waters.

Dr Gúbio and Dr Silvia had to wrestle with a series of headaches. They were thrilled about their discovery but upset by what they felt were affronts. Dr Silvia told me with a note of irony in her voice, "The day after the Zika virus was detected, we went from being two big nobodies to media stars. . . . There was a constant stream of journalists in and out of the lab with their cameras and lights and we couldn't get any work done." While the laboratory's hardships inspired the Brazilian press to portray the two researchers as "heroes" (one magazine ranked them among the "10 heroes of 2015"[49]), the losers of the scientific competition (and there were many) questioned how the couple had acquired the primers and equipment and challenged their ethical and methodological procedures.

"The harshest criticism we received was that we had handled the samples improperly. And that we had imported material without the authorization of Anvisa [essentially equivalent to the US Food and Drug Administration] and hadn't complied with regulations," said Dr Gúbio, his voice choked with resentment. The controversy spilled over into the news, with headlines such as "Diagnoses of Zika cases in Bahia may be wrong."[50] The press also brought up the allegation that the cross-reactivity between the dengue and Zika viruses meant there might be false positives among the Zika results.

The wealthier laboratories of southern Brazil boast the solid structure needed to battle an epidemic or make rapid advances in research. Dr Cláudia works in a laboratory that is part of the Fiocruz public health structure, where engaging in scientific competition and addressing urgent health concerns is routine. She had requested and been granted prior approval from their institution's ethics committee before receiving the samples sent by Dr Kleber. "We have ethics committee approval to receive and work with these samples," she told me. "We're a Fiocruz reference laboratory, Biosafety Level 3."

Just as I had grilled Dr Cláudia about discoverers and timelines, I asked Dr Gúbio about the origin of the primers on more than one occasion. The answer was always the same: the laboratory had been in possession of them since 2014; they had been imported earlier, as part of another batch of research material and in compliance with regulations. I pushed to know how much the discovery of ZIKV in Brazil had cost them. The answer: "Maybe $1,100 to $1,500."

Dr Gúbio sent five of the samples that had tested positive for ZIKV to the government reference laboratory, Evandro Chagas, for confirmation. The kind of testing urged two months earlier by Dr Celso was finally done. This is how Dr Gúbio explained their reason for sending the institute only five of the seven samples: "We held back two because that's the only way we could guarantee our control of the samples we sent in." He was aware that they were in a competition and that it was far from a sure thing that they would be recognized as the discoverers. It was only on May 18, 2015 that the Evandro Chagas Institute issued an official letter, stating that they had confirmed ZIKV in four of the samples from Camaçari. It is worth remembering that the institute belongs to Fiocruz, the same public health foundation that houses Dr Cláudia's lab.

On May 14, 2015, Arthur Chioro, Brazil's then health minister, announced that Zika was circulating in Brazil. He stated at a press conference that day:

> The confirmation came from the Evandro Chagas Institute this morning. We received confirmation for the eight samples that were sent in from Camaçari, Bahia, and eight samples from Rio Grande do Norte, in relation to the Zika virus. But I want to emphasize that the ministry is investigating 1,200 cases of Zika in the Northeast. However, Zika does not worry us. It is a benign disease, which can be cured.[51]

In closing, the minister reiterated that the Ministry of Health was concerned instead with dengue and described the mild symptoms of Zika. There was no reason for the Brazilian public to worry, he insisted.

It was not until June 17, 2015 that the Bahia Department of Health issued a statement in the form of a technical report:

> On April 29, 2015, researchers at the Health Sciences Institute of the Federal University of Bahia (ICS/UFBA) informed the press that they had detected the Zika virus in eight blood samples from patients from the municipality of Camaçari, using real-time RT-PCR. On May 21, the Ministry of Health advised that the methodology used by the researchers had been validated.[52]

The response time of government bureaucracy had not kept pace with the researchers' excitement.

I have no doubt that Dr Gúbio and Dr Silvia were the first to identify the Zika virus circulating in Brazil. The blood samples collected by Dr Antônio provided the key to the right experiment. I cannot say whether the Bahian couple had heard Dr Kleber proclaim to all corners of Brazil that the mysterious illness or allergy was Zika. Dr Gúbio assured me that he had never heard any other physician or scientist raise the Zika hypothesis. According to him, their discovery was rooted in a tight blend of research and spiritual illumination.

Dr Gúbio has been a Spiritist for 30 years. Just as he spent days and nights in the laboratory, following the trail of Dr Antônio's suspicion that there was "more going on here," Dr Gúbio believes he was entrusted with a spiritual mission of discovery. His laboratory had purchased the primers precisely nine months before April 29, 2015. In his words – confided to me almost as if he expected them to be dismissed – the primers were in the laboratory thanks to the "guidance of spiritual interests." For him, a Northeasterner who is not intimidated by notions of so-called scientific neutrality, this was the simple, indisputable reason why their lab possessed the primers for a disease that was then unknown in Brazil. "I'm being honest when I tell you this. How could I have imagined that one day we'd have Zika – and nine months earlier?"

Whether Dr Gúbio heard from the other world, or from Dr Kleber, that Zika was hidden in that blood, one thing is for certain: he and his wife deserve scientific credit for paying heed to the hypothesis and testing it in accordance with scientific protocols. More importantly, these background stories leave it clear that if we had to shape our understanding of the events surrounding the detection of Zika in Brazil solely around the information provided through scientific channels and without the eye-witness testimony of those who traveled the dusty roads of the Northeast drawing blood or who conducted lab tests into the wee hours of the morning, it would be a very different history.

Dr Cláudia's team was the first to have their paper on the isolation of ZIKV released. It was submitted to the journal *Memórias do Instituto Oswaldo Cruz*, a publication of her parent institute, Fiocruz, on May 17, 2015, and accepted for publication one week later, on May 25. Experience from the Ebola epidemic in Africa had alerted academic journals in the health field to the need for more urgent publication in risk situations.[53] Prominent periodicals had accelerated their peer-review and preprint processes so they could inform the scientific community of discoveries in real time. Fiocruz knew the topic was urgent; moreover, one of its own researchers had signed the paper.

Dr Gúbio, Dr Silvia, and Dr Antônio submitted their article to the international journal *Emerging Infectious Diseases* on May 28, 2015, but it underwent editing. The peer reviewers asked that the dengue tests be repeated because they were worried that improper handling might have yielded false positives. The paper only came out in October 2015, five months after publication of the article by the researchers in Paraná.

Both Brazilian and international publications steer shy of assigning primacy. The question matters little to ordinary people who have fallen ill. Researchers, however, are concerned about recognition and possible research benefits. The title of the paper by Dr Cláudia and collaborators made a bold claim: "First report of autochthonous transmission of Zika virus in Brazil."[54]

The version of the paper originally submitted to *Emerging Infectious Diseases* was likewise meant to claim primacy: "The first detection of Zika virus infection in the Americas and its relation to an outbreak of maculopapular rash in Brazil" (in Portuguese). One of the three peer reviewers apparently agreed: "This article presents a major finding: description of the first confirmed cases of infection by Zika virus in the Americas." But the editor wanted nothing to do with this talk in the pages of his journal and so he made them change the title. He wrote:

EID [*Emerging Infectious Diseases*] readers place very low value on claims of primacy. . . . We no longer publish them and routinely delete all such claims in peer review or copyediting.

EID readers are interested in disease emergence into new areas or populations and factors that influence emergence. Craft your next revision (and the title) accordingly, without using the word "first" or similar language implying a claim of primacy.[55]

In this veritable tutorial on what should matter in science's quest for knowledge, the editor makes it clear that he cares little about ranking, recognition, or the sense of achievement felt by researchers from countries on the periphery of global science.

Notwithstanding this lesson in humility from the anonymous editor, I am confident that if Dr Gúbio had not announced their discovery to the press, if he had not let himself be cross-examined by research colleagues and Ministry of Health staff on the days following April 29, 2015, and if his team hadn't sent their samples to the Evandro Chagas Institute for a supplementary round of testing, his name, Dr Antônio's, and Dr. Silvia's would have vanished from the official history of science, since the paper that came out first was written by the second group to isolate the virus. The most fascinating thing about how science constructs the images of its heroes and other figures is the fact that the two teams of laboratory scientists only threw themselves into the race for discovery because they were nudged to do so by bedside physicians, who worked alongside them: Dr Kleber, in Rio Grande do Norte; Dr Celso, in Alagoas; and Dr Antônio, in Bahia.

As understandable as it is that Dr Cláudia lauded Dr Kleber's wisdom in identifying Zika even before her primers had handed down a verdict, there were other clinicians who had entertained the same suspicion. Maybe the reason neither Dr Celso, Dr Antônio, nor anyone else played the same proactive role as Dr Kleber or displayed as much persistence in pursuing the ZIKV hypothesis was that they were not as well trained to anticipate the arrival of the virus in Brazil. And that brings me back to the images of mutilated bodies and ex-votos, to legs seared by pain, to the itchy skin of those people from the Northeast – the very first people to be troubled by this peculiar viral illness, and who turned to drugstores and doctors in hopes of finding remedies and answers.

The Evandro Chagas Institute detected Zika in four samples from Camaçari, three from women and one from a man. Neither Dr Gúbio nor Dr Antônio knows anything more about these people than their gender and age. The need to erase any personal identification reduced them to nothing but blood samples for use in investigating the mystery illness. Nor does Dr Celso remember the names or stories behind the body parts captured in his photographs of rashes and conjunctivitis. Dr Kleber is a story-teller, but he also talks about the sick in group terms. The fact of the matter is that not even the stricken individuals who enabled a major discovery in the first chapter of Brazil's Zika epidemic know that they were the ones who offered pieces of their bodies to science. They are anonymous Northeasterners.

# THE FIRST GENERATION OF WOMEN

## THE FOREIGNER

Sofia Tezza is a young Italian whose heart moved her to Brazil. She married a Brazilian and was already pregnant when she realized things weren't going to work out between them. With help from her parents, she practically fled back to Italy. She holds no hard feelings about this period; she just misses the three nameless kittens that kept her company. She remembers her days with Zika; her skin was on fire and not even a cold bath could soothe the little bumps all over her body. When she called her doctor, she heard exactly what other first-generation mothers-to-be heard from their doctors during the Zika epidemic in Brazil: "Don't worry. It's nothing. Just a virus. It'll go away in three or four days. You don't need to take anything." So she took no medication. She stayed home with her cats, dividing her time between travel preparations and goodbyes. Before she left, she had another prenatal ultrasound, the first one after her rash. The doctor's playful prediction would eventually prove true but not in the way she had intended it: "This boy is going to be a handful."

Sofia left Brazil when she was six months pregnant, taking with her the exams that showed a dancing boy, Pietro the Great. Sofia arrived back in Italy on August 1, 2015, a hot summer day. Her father wanted his grandson to grow up around the family. The first ultrasound in Italy showed a different image. It was as if she were looking at a negative of what she'd seen before. Pietro's brain was covered with white patches. And he was resting more every day.

"She's young and can have 30 kids," the Italian doctor told Sofia's mother. Sofia went mute, and her mother became the voice that questioned doctors and lamented the senselessness of this unknown disease. The doctor explained that Pietro's brain had been compromised; she said she'd never seen anything like it in her entire career. Sofia set off on a pilgrimage to the offices of prominent doctors, some of whom were more foreign than she had been in Brazil. They were all just as dumbfounded as the first European doctor who had visualized her baby. "They'd never seen anything like it," she told me. They said her child would be "a vegetable," a metaphor that gets caught in Sofia's throat.

Sofia began researching. She had to discover what science had not yet, and so she became a scientist of her own body. Something had happened to Pietro. If it was a new disease, Sofia wanted to name it and know it, so she could care for her child better. She scoured the news from Brazil but there was no talk of any illness that affected fetuses, just talk of the spreading Zika epidemic in the precise region of Northeast Brazil where she had lived. Nothing and nobody could explain why Pietro grew quieter every day.

Sofia traveled to Slovenia, site of a renowned center for tropical diseases. She was eight months pregnant but her belly had stopped growing. Pietro was even smaller than the images on the ultrasound taken after Sofia's skin had recovered from the rash. At the University Medical Center in Ljubljana, she found her final answers; there would be no cure or treatment for Pietro. And the doctors there were just as astonished as all the others by the serious damage done to the baby's brain.

The details recorded in the official history of science differ from those stored in Sofia's flesh-and-blood memory. According to the scientists who studied her case, labor was induced to terminate the pregnancy. Sofia told me Pietro died naturally and labor was only induced after he had stopped dancing in her belly. I didn't confront her with the version found in "Zika Virus Associated with Microcephaly," the article by the researchers from Slovenia.[1] Sofia also read the paper, which was the first publication in the history of medicine to report the detection of Zika virus DNA in a fetus – and which also reported that the woman had asked for an abortion.[2] The paper received international coverage, making a significant contribution to the second chapter of the Zika epidemic in Brazil.[3] As science heralded a major discovery, a grieving woman mourned her child.

## THE NORTHEASTERNERS

It was in the parched rural region of Paraíba that I had my first contact with women who had caught Zika during their pregnancies. Some had recently given birth and were busy with their tiny babies; others were mourning the death of their newborns. One of them was Géssica Eduardo dos Santos, resident of Juazeirinho, a town with a population of some 16,000. Géssica is married to Silvandro da Silva Lima and has a daughter named Samara. She got pregnant with her second in April 2015, this time hoping for a boy. When she was 20 weeks along, she paid out of pocket for an anatomy scan so she could learn the baby's sex. "I noticed the doctor got strange during the exam, so I asked her: Is my baby all right?" The answer laid Géssica's original plans to rest. She began living with a feeling of despair that hasn't left her since.

The family inhabits a brightly painted little house typical of this area of Northeast Brazil. The windows are small and its low tile roof has no underlayment, bare rafters visible from inside. The family uses water stored in buckets and barrels to wash their clothes, take baths, and cook because they don't always have running water. Like many streets in Juazeirinho, theirs is unpaved and always dusty. Géssica, 25, spends her time being a mother, going to mass, and visiting relatives. There's no air-conditioning in a town where the power goes out all the time, and the mosquito netting that she and her husband sleep under had failed to do its job. A few blocks away from Géssica's, there is no sanitation at all and mosquitoes of all varieties abound.

Given the unexpected results of her first ultrasound, Géssica and her husband decided to head to Campina Grande, the healthcare hub for dozens of small towns in rural Paraíba. It was there that she met Dr Adriana Melo, who would later go from being an unknown specialist in fetal medicine in what is one of the poorer states in Northeast Brazil to being a name in the pages of international science journals.

It was November 2015. By then, everyone knew that the new disease among them was Zika and not some run-of-the-mill viral illness, allergy, or mild dengue. What nobody knew yet was that Zika could harm fetal development. During Géssica's ultrasound, Dr Adriana told her as gently as possible that the situation was serious; the image showed that "the fetus was accumulating fluid and a part of the cerebellum was missing." By that time, Dr Adriana was growing alarmed by what she was seeing in her private practice in fetal medicine. Microcephaly with intracranial calcifications is rare, but over the previous month, she had presented this same diagnosis to three other women besides Géssica. Every one of them had said they had come down with a bug during pregnancy. She was hearing similar reports of babies born with microcephaly from her colleagues in the neighboring state of Pernambuco. Dr Adriana was the first to sit up and take notice of this development during pregnancy.

Some weeks earlier, another woman from Juazeirinho, Maria da Conceição Alcantara Oliveira Matias – Conceição for short – had been in her office. Géssica and Conceição didn't know each other, but doctors in rural Paraíba had started recommending that their patients consult with Dr Adriana because she was a specialist in intracranial calcifications. Conceição and her husband, Mário Matias Maracajá Filho, wanted this baby very much. They'd been married five years and for the last one had been trying to get pregnant. At the age of 34, Conceição was in a hurry to become a mother. She did some tests and prepared herself for the pregnancy, which came in June, the month Paraíba celebrates the Feast of St John. The Feast is more than a holy day in rural Paraíba; the year is divided into before and after June 24. On the eve of the event, her body ached; she had no interest whatsoever in the festivities. The next day, Conceição had pain in her joints and was covered with red bumps. She went to a public clinic to see if it was mild dengue. They drew her blood, and the doctor assured her it wasn't dengue. He said the illness had its own name: Zika. It was June 2015 and Conceição was in the seventh week of her first pregnancy. Her hands wouldn't close, as if the joints of her fingers refused to obey her. The red spots vanished as quickly as they'd appeared but the body aches stayed with her for a good while.

Conceição's husband accompanied her to Dr Adriana's office. He was excited about becoming a father. He stood by his wife's side, filming the first exam, which showed they were expecting a girl. Perhaps because he was so excited, Mário didn't notice when happiness drained out of the room. Dr Adriana had turned off the screen and Conceição was crying. She was 22 weeks along and didn't need an ultrasound technician to point out the white spots that were now mottling her baby's brain. Conceição said many thoughts ran through her head as the image on the screen burned into her memory: "Nothing had gone wrong with my pregnancy. Everything was planned. I didn't travel the first months. I didn't eat seafood. I didn't do a bunch of things so I wouldn't get an infection. I couldn't figure it out." All Conceição could think about were the children she worked with as a physical therapist. "What would those calcifications do to my daughter? I was afraid of what might be coming."

Dr Adriana ordered the tests repeated every 20 days. Conceição found every appointment extremely distressing. She could never sleep the night before and Dr Adriana's waiting room was, in the doctor's own words, "like death row, mothers awaiting their sentence." At each new exam, further changes appeared. Conceição and her husband began studying on their own. They read whatever they could and pored over images of other children with microcephaly. And every day at the public healthcare clinic where she worked, Conceição suffered alone as she watched the children, thinking to herself that her daughter might very well be like them. That's when she decided to talk to her obstetrician. "The only thing I had was Zika," she told him. The doctor didn't reject the hypothesis, but still, he preferred to play it safe: "Zika is a new disease. There's no way of saying."

Dr Adriana was in contact with the general practitioners and specialists who belonged to the WhatsApp group "CHIKV, the mission," where there was a steady exchange of messages about the triple epidemic of dengue, chikungunya, and Zika. Around the same time, the city of Recife announced to the nation that it was witnessing a sharp surge in the number of newborns with microcephaly. And the Zika epidemic continued its march. There were worries about the possible causal agent of the microcephaly: dengue, chikungunya, or Zika, or maybe an infection like toxoplasmosis or cytomegalovirus (CMV).[4] Two neuropediatricians in Recife, Ana Van der Linden and her daughter Vanessa, had started noticing an increase in babies born with a peculiar kind of microcephaly. The pattern of calcifications was also strange. At first they suspected CMV, but the white spots on the brains were unlike any they'd seen before.[5] Dr Adriana had been struck by the images of Conceição's baby and had compared them to Géssica's. The patterns of calcifications and brain damage were different but in both cases there was something typical of the anatomical changes caused by an infection. Like Dr Ana and Dr Vanessa, Dr Adriana also suspected CMV, although the white spots were more destructive of the brain than what is observed with the latter.

On November 14, 2015, Géssica, Conceição, and their husbands flew to São Paulo, where Dr Adriana had arranged for an international scientist to analyze their ultrasound images and offer diagnoses. A few days before they left, Dr Adriana had collected amniotic fluid from both women and sent it to the Fiocruz reference laboratory in Rio de Janeiro, where it would be tested for the presence of Zika. Conceição felt stronger than Géssica. For over a month, she had been studying how the intracranial calcifications and microcephaly might impact her daughter. Time had alleviated some of her sorrow; so too had her daily contact with other children whose development depended heavily on specialized care. But Géssica had received her diagnosis just over one week earlier.

Upon their arrival in São Paulo, the women repeated several exams and filled out seemingly endless questionnaires. The results confirmed what Conceição and Géssica already knew. Worse, they had to hear the news through an interpreter, because the doctor from abroad didn't speak Portuguese. Just as complicated as putting words to one's pain is not knowing how those words will reach the ears of someone who has the power to provide health care and hand down a sentence.

The foreign specialist told Géssica her case was very serious. "He said it wasn't simple," she remembers. "The odds were very bad. [My baby] might die shortly after birth, or he might end up a vegetable in the NICU." An invisible virus was destroying her son's brain, yet for someone who had eagerly been expecting a baby, for someone who had decided to replace science with prayer, "vegetable" was a word as unbearable to her as it had been to Sofia. Watching Géssica's case unfold, Conceição realized there was a difference between them: "They said my baby had a good chance of surviving, that she might be normal. But Géssica's baby was a more serious case. He'd be a vegetable."

They returned to Juazeirinho. Géssica resolved to live out the rest of her pregnancy. "I decided not to cry anymore. I decided to enjoy my pregnancy." Conceição armed herself with manuals and read up on early stimulation. On Tuesday, November 17, the day after Dr Adriana told the two women that Zika had been isolated from their amniotic fluid, Conceição saw herself on television, one of "two pregnant women from Paraíba." She didn't need to watch anymore; she knew it was Géssica and her.[6] Conceição closed herself off. She wanted nothing to do with being an expert in rashes or suffering. She felt it should be the doctors who talked to the press. "I'm not going to go around talking about my pain," she said. Géssica, on the other hand, opened herself up to the world. She told her story until it grieved her. It was a long story, and it bothered her that the journalists seemed to latch on to only minor details. When I met Géssica, two weeks after the birth and death of her son João Guilherme, it was the first time she'd resumed talking after a period of self-imposed silence. She insisted on showing me the nursery closet where her mourning was locked up among baby clothes and booties. "When I miss him, I come here to smell his things. I imagine what it would be like, him wearing these clothes."

Conceição's and Géssica's stories ran parallel through the end of their pregnancies: the day Catarina Maria was born, João Guilherme died. It was February 5, 2016. Géssica tells the story of the birth as best her memory permits; she fell asleep immediately after her son was born and only the next day had the chance to cradle him for a few minutes.[7] João Guilherme passed away moments later.

Dr Adriana's sister, Dr Fabiana Melo, is an obstetrician in residence. The young doctor tells a different version of this story, and she cries whenever she thinks back on it: "Géssica saw her son, but then she dropped off to sleep. We knew she wouldn't remember, so at the family's request, the baby was resuscitated." And so João

Guilherme survived a night in the neonatal intensive care unit, where Géssica remembers "doing everything a mother wants to do with a child. I smelled him, I rocked him until I said goodbye, even after he'd passed away."

Géssica and Conceição were the first two women in Brazil's Zika saga to donate amniotic fluid, enabling researchers to discover that the virus crosses the placenta.[8] Géssica went further. With the burning grief of someone who held her baby for only a few brief moments, she offered him to science. While still in the hospital, she authorized the medical team to remove from her dead son's body whatever was needed for scientific research. It was Dr Fabiana, apprentice obstetrician and practitioner of humanized childbirth, who carried the baby in her arms to be immortalized by science. Géssica explained what she did in these words: "I didn't want to be selfish, with all the mothers in the world not having an answer."

Like Dr Adriana, Conceição and Géssica were women from rural Paraíba who were unknown to science or scientists but who managed to ask the right questions at moments of great personal anguish. Sofia buried Pietro in October 2015 and dreams of him in the company of other babies in heaven. After Catarina Maria's birth in February 2016, Conceição made her daughter's body an extension of hers, working to stimulate her baby beyond anything the manuals call for. Géssica held onto João Guilherme's baby things for a long time, until she found a mother whose newborn son was much like hers, and then she gave away her dreams. She never tires of looking at the photo of her son, who died in the hospital. Alessandra de Sousa Amorim, mother to Samuel and four girls, happily accepted João Guilherme's baby things. She is married to Alexandre Oliveira Santiago and lives in Pedregal, a neighborhood of Campina Grande. They are just a few of the women from the first generation of Brazil's Zika epidemic.

I also heard the stories of Adilma, Adriana, Alane, Alda, Aldayane, Aldenora, Alessandra, Amanda, Ana Angélica, Ana Carolina, Antônia Vitória, Arlene, Cileneide, Conceição, Cristiane, Edna Cinthia, Edna de Lira, Ellen, Evitevargas, Francicleide, Francileide, Francinelma, Gislene, Helena, Ianka, Inês, Izabel, Josefa Juliene, Josiane, Josimary, Josivânia, Juliana Josina, Kalissandra, Leonora, Lívia, Lizandra, Luana, Maria Carolina, Maria Germana, Maria José, Mirian, Nelsa, Olânia, Raquel, Rosilda, Sabrina, Sayonara, Vanicleide, and Yasmin.[9] All of them live in rural Paraíba and travel hours in their efforts to discover in their children what science does not yet know.

# FOOTPRINTS OF
# THE VIRUS

## THE PARALYZING SYNDROME

By late April 2015, word was out that Zika was assailing Brazil. But newspaper headlines continued to report that people with symptoms of mild dengue were flooding emergency services. Correct identification of the virus behind the symptoms remained a challenge. Dr Carlos Brito set about trying to figure out who was suffering from what in Recife's emergency rooms, especially since the triple epidemic of dengue, chikungunya, and Zika might be camouflaging other arboviruses as well. "Although the Zika hypothesis is stronger, this study will also consider the chikungunya, Oropouche, and Mayaro viruses and even a variation of some types of dengue," he explained to reporters when asked about the new initiative to monitor the sick in Recife.[1] The list of arboviruses repeated by the press read like a table out of Sir Patrick Manson's manual on tropical medicine.

The six months from May to October 2015 brought further information on the new illness. People began showing up at emergency rooms because they had developed a form of paralysis. Children and adults, some of them elderly, all experienced similar symptoms. The malady became known as the "paralyzing syndrome." The patient would present a milder version of the pain and itching typical of Zika, but then her body would suddenly quit obeying. Not the whole body, just parts of it – Dr Celso's ex-votos had apparently now lost their will to move.[2] Medicine had long had a name for this new ailment: Guillain-Barré syndrome, first described in the literature in 1916.[3]

GBS is one of the most common types of neurological emergencies but few people appreciate how serious it is. About 20 percent of those who contract it continue to have symptoms for the rest of their lives, and 5 percent die of it.[4] In 2012, the prestigious *New England Journal of Medicine* published a review article on the diagnosis and treatment of GBS. The study looked at 85 sources, but nowhere did it mention the hypothesis that Zika might set off the syndrome.[5]

Medical literature first examined the possibility of a relation between Zika and this immune-mediated neurological process following the outbreak in French Polynesia, which ran from late 2013 to 2014. These initial articles were essentially case reports; in other words, they presented information that had been gathered at the bedside. The earliest was published in March 2014 and describes a patient in French Polynesia.[6] In July 2014, a more thoroughgoing study analyzed blood samples from the sentinel health surveillance network in the South Pacific country and pinpointed 40 cases of GBS. Exercising scientific caution, researchers kept their statements timid at that point: "The direct involvement of the ZIKV . . . still needs to be investigated because of prolonged co-circulation of the dengue and Zika viruses."[7] Evidence in support of a causal relationship between Zika and GBS was still scant in 2015, so it is no surprise that physicians on the other side of the planet were oblivious to the possibility.

The so-called paralyzing syndrome surfaced in Brazil around the same time that Zika was detected. The terms "causality" and "correlation" were bandied about in the press and scientific circles, even among physicians who had little to do with epidemiological research. Was this merely a correlation without a causal relationship? That is, were Zika and GBS occurring simultaneously, without any direct link between them?[8] This kind of mix-up is easy, especially when a new disease shows up at the same time that a new virus is found circulating. And it seemed simple enough to argue that Zika causes GBS. Residents of Camaçari, in Bahia, had followed much the same logic: because they lived near a polluting industry, they quickly assumed that the mysterious new illness was triggered by contaminated water. But although pollution causes many diseases, this wasn't the case in Camaçari; the public had simply fallen prey to fallacious reasoning.[9]

WhatsApp remained an agile tool for exchanging information on the baffling new cases. The "CHIKV, the mission" group was quieter, but Dr Brito initiated other correspondence. Two fellow neurologists, Dr Maria Iris de Morais Machado and Dr Maria Lucia Brito (no relation), helped him survey cases of GBS. On May 15, 2015, the women notified him that they were seeing patients whose neurological symptoms had been preceded by dengue. The neurologists also reported that cases were up five times over the previous year. Donning his two hats, clinician and epidemiologist, Dr Brito went to the hospital to interview each patient in person. It wasn't dengue; it was Zika. His colleagues in neurology were not yet familiar with the pattern of the novel virus. He checked each new patient with paralysis for prior symptoms of Zika; his numbers did not stop growing. Dr Brito and a group of bedside physicians initiated a study to monitor GBS cases. In June 2015, five of seven patients whose cerebrospinal fluid had been proven to contain ZIKV were diagnosed with GBS.[10]

Dr Brito had gained a reputation as the fellow who kept pestering physicians of all specialties for the latest news, and once again his clinical and epidemiological nose was sensing something in the air. The virus had been given a name and *Aedes aegypti* was known to be its nasty vector. Now the doctor's fight expanded into showing that the hosts of cases that epidemiological surveillance was attributing to dengue were actually Zika. Dr Brito's voice still rises a notch when he recalls the recommendation handed down by the Pernambuco Department of Health: suspected cases

with a hypothetical diagnosis of ZIKV shall be tied, for the purposes of epidemiological surveillance, to a suspicion of dengue and reported to the Reportable Diseases Surveillance System (SINAN), Dengue Online. This measure is meant to guide spatial monitoring of transmission of the virus for the purposes of vector control, an action common to both illnesses.[11]

As a result, from the time that Zika was found to be circulating in Brazil until October 10, 2015, the epidemiological report issued by Pernambuco – one of the epicenters of Zika in Brazil – tallied only four cases of ZIKV infection, as confirmed by the Evandro Chagas Institute.[12]

As Dr Brito saw it, the epidemiological surveillance figures effectively muddled the three epidemics. He insisted on explaining something basic about clinical practice to me: "Once an epidemic has been confirmed, diagnosis is clinical. The laboratory is only used in critical cases." A physician's clinical skills would thus be essential in differentiating the three epidemics and ensuring that epidemiological surveillance had accurate numbers on the circulating viruses and could offer proper guidance. Because the numbers were such a mess, Dr Brito was even more surprised when Dr Vanessa Van der Linden, the neuropediatrician from Recife, called him on the afternoon of October 19, 2015 to talk about children with microcephaly.

## THE NEUROPEDIATRICIANS FROM RECIFE

Dr Vanessa Van der Linden and her mother, Dr Ana Van der Linden, are prominent practitioners of pediatric neurology who often put their heads together in their work, approaching it as in the spirit of medicine, where, as Dr Ana puts it, "cases always come in pairs." The fact that both mother and daughter opted for this specialization is surprising not only because it pays poorly in Brazil but also because the workload is doubled, since a pediatrician always has two patients in the office: mother and child.

Dr Vanessa grows emotional when she remembers her encounter with the baby she calls patient zero: "I can't forget [him]. The case was unlike anything I'd ever seen before." The term "patient zero" is somewhat problematic. When used in reference to a disease that is transmitted vertically, like Zika, patient zero might very well refer to the mother who caught the virus as much as to the newborn affected by it. If there is a true patient zero for Brazil's Zika epidemic, she might best be found among the women who fell ill during their pregnancy, like Géssica Eduardo dos Santos, Maria da Conceição Alcantara Oliveira Matias, and Sofia Tezza.

Dr Vanessa doesn't begin her story with the women, since her specialty is children. Her patient zero was one of a set of twins. The mother has never spoken publicly about the matter; what we know of her story has come through her husband, who identified himself only as P.J. to the press. He told the BBC: "I remembered that in December, when she had this rash all over her body, our town in rural Pernambuco was one of those with the most cases of dengue in the state. Then that feeling hit me: 'Gosh, we could have prevented it'."[13] Back then, Zika was still a nameless viral illness, at best confused with dengue in the Brazilian Northeast. Doctors would later rely on women's memories of pain and itching to recover their histories of Zika during pregnancy.

Dr Vanessa saw the twin in her private office. The baby didn't show any symptoms that the Zika virus was in its blood, like red bumps or swollen joints. Instead, he was a portrait of the destruction that Zika can leave in a newborn's brain. The visit took place in the first week of August 2015. At that time nothing in the scientific literature contained the slightest hint that the Zika virus could cross the placenta and damage fetal development. Dr Vanessa turned to what she knew about viruses and infections, searching the medical manuals for information on excessive scalp skin and especially on severe microcephaly. Recalling her diagnosis from that first visit, she says she found the pattern of calcifications very peculiar, because they were "extensive and symmetrical"; the excess skin suggested a "sudden intrauterine reduction of the brain during development."

The brothers were fraternal twins, each with its own placenta, and the virus had affected only one of them. But the doctor had no reason to suspect Zika.

As a physician, Dr Vanessa looked at the twin precisely as medicine had taught her. "Microcephaly is only a sign, not a diagnosis," she told me on several occasions. So when she investigated the newborn's case, that is precisely how she viewed his microcephaly: a sign of something else. Her initial hypothesis was cytomegalovirus (CMV). When dozens of tests came back negative, she moved to genetic disorders. The family had private health insurance and could afford the exams required by her hunt for a diagnosis. Dr Vanessa often discusses difficult cases with a colleague, Dr Regina Coeli Ramos, who advised her to test the baby for chikungunya. The test was only available at a private laboratory and not covered by any insurance plan. The baby's father weighed the cost and decided against it.

As much as the signs presented by the twin were challenging to diagnose, Dr Vanessa didn't think it was anything other than a difficult case at first. But while she continued studying her patient, she also visited public hospitals in Recife, as part of her daily routine. On September 15, the twin turned out to have company. When Dr Vanessa arrived at the hospital where she worked, the medical team awaited her with startling news: three newborns in the maternity ward displayed microcephaly. She spent some time with the infants, once again noting the peculiar calcifications and excessive scalp skin. "Their CT-scans were very typical," she explained. In medicine, the question is always "typical of what," and in this case the pediatrician meant typical of a sickness caused by infection. She was convinced it wasn't CMV; something strange was going on. She had already eliminated syphilis, HIV, and toxoplasmosis in the twin. Through a battery of tests she advanced into the unknown, beyond the relatively obvious hypotheses suggested by her colleagues. She decided to call Dr Ana. "Mom, something's wrong."

Dr Ana listened intently to her daughter. Three cases in one maternity ward was astonishing. Pernambuco had recorded a total of ten cases of microcephaly in 2013 and 12 in 2014.[14] Dr Ana decided to make her own expedition through Recife's hospitals, where she is highly respected in her field. She has been a professor at the Federal University of Pernambuco for many years, and a good number of today's neuropediatricians in Recife were once her students. In one afternoon at a single hospital, she saw seven children with microcephaly. She was on the phone to her daughter in a flash: "Vanessa, I'm here at the hospital and there are seven babies with microcephaly. Their heads aren't any different from one another; they're all very much alike." This information was enough to prompt Dr Ana, Dr Vanessa, and Dr Regina to set up a specialized microcephaly clinic. Dr Vanessa sent a WhatsApp message to fellow neuropediatricians at the ten or so other public hospitals in Recife and asked that any newborn with microcephaly be referred to it. At first, she heard back from only one resident: "I have a case, but it's cytomegalovirus."

Dr Ana and Dr Vanessa pressed on. They visited hospitals in person and asked that cases be referred to them. At one place, Dr Ana organized the wards to facilitate the diagnosis of newborns with microcephaly. "We have five wards . . . each of which can receive six to eight mothers and their babies. Three of them were almost filled with children with microcephaly," Dr Ana told me. The doctors had originally expected the clinic to receive ten infants.

Mother and daughter were both certain that a new infectious disease was on the loose. The challenge was identifying the pathogenic agent. The mothers told stories of falling ill during pregnancy, their bodies covered with rashes. The twin's mother told her doctor: "I had the itches, like everybody else. They just lasted a day." The trio of pediatricians decided to look for help. If these clinical features were indeed indicative of a congenital infection, it was essential to discover which viruses had been circulating in the homes of the women in the first half of 2015, when they had become pregnant.

Dr Adélia Souza is a neuropediatrician and a colleague of Dr Vanessa's. She listened attentively to the story of the twins and the other cases at the newly inaugurated clinic, paying close attention to the symptoms reported by the women and the clinical signs in newborns. Dr Vanessa told her firmly: "I've tested and have laboratory proof for everything I know of." She decided to go straight to the Pernambuco Department of Health and, on October 14, 2015, she had an audience with the secretary, Dr José Iran Costa Júnior. She told him of her concerns and suspicions and asked for help with funding; unless she could run further tests, she could not verify her suspicion that a virus was circulating and possibly causing microcephaly. She recounted the story of the twin and the clinic that was receiving dozens of newborns with microcephaly. Costa Júnior reportedly contacted epidemiological surveillance and asked for records on newborns from all maternity wards in Pernambuco.

Dr Vanessa was even more concerned after this meeting. Dr Adélia suggested she discuss it with Dr Brito. "He's looking into this," she explained. "He's researching the effects of arboviruses in Recife." Dr Vanessa followed her colleague's suggestion and phoned

Dr Brito; the two physicians spoke for nearly two hours. Dr Brito was convinced that the piece of the puzzle identified by Dr Vanessa revealed the power of the Zika virus; throngs of people had fallen sick in the first few months of 2015, the "paralyzing syndrome" had hit in the middle of the year, and now came the affected newborns. The microcephaly epidemic apparently had been triggered when women were struck by Zika during pregnancy; the cycle seemed to be closing.

As a clinician, Dr Brito once again had to see the sick for himself and so he visited public maternity wards in Recife. As a neuropediatrician, Dr Vanessa turned her attention to arboviruses. It was a "meeting of two minds," they each told me. Over the phone, they agreed to be cautious and not speak to the press until they had advanced in their research. They would stay in constant touch but would follow different paths in their investigations.

Dr Brito tried to persuade his fellow epidemiologists that the microcephaly was not a product of previous underreporting or some genetic factor. He believed they were witnessing a change in an epidemiological pattern, and the cause was the Zika virus. In his view, only someone who had never seen a newborn harmed by Zika could think it boiled down to underreporting. "It was extreme microcephaly," Dr Brito says of what confronted him at the hospitals.[15] Dr Vanessa's patient zero had a head circumference of only 27 cm.

Even if microcephaly had historically been underreported in Pernambuco, Dr Brito was confident this was different. As Dr Vanessa said, microcephaly was a sign but not the only one.[16] Some of the newborns she had seen had normal head circumferences but disproportionate faces. They urgently needed to gather proof right at the hospitals. Dr Brito needed data confirming that Recife was recording a surge in microcephaly and that the mothers had contracted Zika during gestation. The day after his talk with Dr Vanessa, he met with Dr Jucielle Menezes, chief of neonatology at a top hospital in Recife.

Dr Jucielle showed him 16 children with microcephaly that morning; coincidentally, all were Dr Ana's patients. Dr Brito then headed into the field to do a rapid assessment of maternity wards across the state. He drew up a questionnaire, met with mothers, asked them questions, and listened to their stories. This was the first research survey on microcephaly and Zika virus in Brazil. Within a week, Dr Brito had collected stories from 26 women. All of them reported having suffered rashes, itchiness, and aches and pains during pregnancy. All had in fact caught Zika during pregnancy but thought it was a viral illness or maybe a mild case of dengue.

Dr Brito keeps a picture of some of these mothers as they gathered in a room. "An unforgettable photo" is how he describes it. It is a candid shot, no planning, no careful set-up. People aren't looking at the camera because nobody is celebrating anything. The photo shows people crowded into a miniscule space where a lot is happening. Six women hold their tiny babies. You cannot see the tracks left by the virus, because the newborns are swaddled in blankets or colorful pajamas. Some of the mothers exchange glances; others stare off into space. One of them is wearing a green hospital gown; maybe she went straight from the ward to the survey room. Women in white coats move about the room, writing answers down on clipboards. If we were to put a face on the Zika virus at the moment that science first confronted the possibility of vertical transmission, it would be found in this photo: anonymous women, hospital wristbands on their arms and newborns in them.

Dr Brito felt he had to expand his clinical observations. He thought the numbers justified a public health alert, but he decided to call Dr Kleber Luz, the physician who had first believed the Zika virus was on the loose in Brazil. Dr Kleber remembers their conversation and his ensuing worry. "I don't know anything," he told his colleague. "Give me 48 hours to see if I can find data on microcephaly here." He thought of Sofia Tezza as he hung up. One month earlier, he had replied to her anxious queries. He put off re-reading her email, leery of what he might have missed. He cancelled all of his other commitments and launched the second survey on microcephaly in Brazil, starting with his fellow pediatricians. His question was straightforward: "Have you seen any children with microcephaly?" The answer was "yes." There were indeed more cases of the disorder, but he heard no reports of Zika among the mothers.

Dr Kleber asked his colleagues for their patients' phone numbers and then called them one by one. "It wasn't easy," he recalls. "The poor women – a baby with a small head, postpartum. They were worried about other things. They weren't the least bit interested in a survey, in a doctor's interview." Some described the itching and pain they'd felt for a few days while pregnant; others said they hadn't been sick at all during their pregnancy and then they simply cut off the conversation. Dr Kleber could hear the distress in their voices, as their babies wailed in the background. He didn't detect as many cases as in Recife, and he still wasn't convinced. He finally went back to Sofia's email. There it all was, in writing: the calcifications, the hypothesis of a congenital infection, the red bumps and itching during early pregnancy.[17]

Re-reading the Italian woman's email left a bitter taste in Dr Kleber's mouth because he realized he had failed to hear what she was saying. Then phone calls started coming in from the mothers of women who had hurriedly hung up on him. "Doctor, I'm calling to tell you my daughter had Zika. She itched all over. Everybody at home got the itches."[18] In one morning, he learned of 12 women who had caught Zika and whose children were born with small heads. Dr Kleber couldn't stop thinking about Sofia. Before a single physician had paused to reflect, that woman in a distant land had asked the right question: "Doctor, does this disease cause malformation to the fetus?" He called his friend Dr Brito and presented his data. Reviving his participation in "CHIKV, the mission," he sent off two photos of a newborn and wrote: "The cases have begun. Blood tests all negative . . . normal karyotype . . . mother had Zika."[19] It was October 21, 2015.

The figures from Recife and Natal gave Dr Brito the confidence to fast track everything. On October 26, about a week after his conversation with Dr Vanessa, he chaired a meeting of the Pernambuco Regional Board of Medicine (CREMEPE), where he introduced the hypothesis that the Zika virus causes microcephaly. Two days before the meeting, the press had reported that there might be a relation between the virus and microcephaly; Dr Adélia, the same neurologist who had urged Dr Vanessa to speak with Dr Brito, told the interviewer: "It's important to stress that we cannot draw any relation with dengue, chikungunya, or Zika yet. What's happening is that since the beginning of the year, we've been experiencing a dengue epidemic, which has coincided with the gestational period of women who recently had babies with microcephaly."[20] The hypothesis was out there: the Zika virus *might cause* microcephaly. Use of the conditional tense reflected scientific caution, because the possibility of a false correlation had not been wholly discarded.

The meeting of the Regional Board of Medicine was far from a smooth one. The story had leaked to the press and the topic could have complicated ramifications for public health policy in Pernambuco. Furthermore, it had been announced via "CHIKV, the mission" that representatives of the Ministry of Health and the Pan American Health Organization (PAHO) would attend, signaling that the subject matter was delicate and should be taken seriously. However, the state specialists who were also expected did not show up. They were offended that the elite forces in health had been included, whereas they had never received a direct invitation; they didn't even know what was going to be discussed, they complained. Dr Brito explained that no official invitation had been extended to anyone. "It was just a closed scientific meeting," he said. But there was no fixing the damage. A byproduct of the meeting was a lasting atmosphere of hard feelings between state specialists and the physician, who was no longer to take part in local government policymaking on Zika or microcephaly.

On October 27, 2015, the Board of Medicine created a Microcephaly Advisory Council. In a report on the new board's epidemiological concerns, an online news service stated: "Records from the Live Birth Information System (SINASC) show that from January through September, 20 babies with this abnormality in brain growth were born in Pernambuco. There have also been 26 new cases of microcephaly in babies born in the past 15 days at public maternity wards."[21] Dr Brito was named coordinator of the medical board's Advisory Council, the first task force to monitor the growth of microcephaly in Brazil.

Meanwhile, Dr Vanessa pressed forward with her research. The mother–daughter duo of neuropediatricians exchanged information almost daily. With every additional newborn reported and referred to their clinic, the words "microcephaly is only one sign" weighed heavier in the air.[22] Along with Dr Regina, the two doctors amassed notes on how overall fetal development was affected. The faces of these babies were disproportionately wide in comparison to their small heads. Many of them displayed "redundant scalp skin," the term for folds of extra skin under the hair and a sign that the skin continues growing after brain development has been interrupted; it is also a sign not observed with other congenital infections. What was originally interpreted as mere fussiness or irritability became understood as part of a condition that included tremors and convulsions. Some babies had dysphagia, that is, trouble eating. In many cases, their hands and feet were contracted, a birth defect called arthrogryposis. Without knowing it, the three doctors were recording the manifestations of an as-yet-unnamed congenital syndrome in the first generation of children harmed by the epidemic.[23]

In addition to the signs apparent on clinical exam, the tomographies of hundreds of newborns revealed the same calcification pattern as the twin who Dr Vanessa called patient zero. One of the news reports on the twin featured a photograph of Dr Ana and Dr Vanessa along with head CT-scans described as from babies affected by ZIKV.[24] It is unusual to see something as technical as a radiological image reproduced in a news report but, as Dr Vanessa put it, the scars from the infection were evident even to the untrained. A thick white band running just underneath the skull appears to wrap the brain in a layer of white rubber. This is not a protective coating but rather the image of calcifications – the scars left by the passage of the virus.

Science had raised many questions, and scientists felt these begged the proclamation of a public health emergency. Physicians in Recife were convinced this was an epidemic of microcephaly; they also felt confident of the tie between Zika and the observed fetal anomalies. But just as any false correlation had to be disproved in the first chapter of Zika, the testimonies of Dr Brito and Dr Vanessa were not enough to sway either policymakers, physicians in southern Brazil, or the international community, by then closely attuned to events in Northeast Brazil.

On November 17, 2015, news came out of Campina Grande, Paraíba, that the obstetrician Dr Adriana Melo had isolated ZIKV from the amniotic fluid of two local women – Géssica and Conceição. Here was the first proof that the Zika virus crosses the placenta and could affect a fetus.

## THE DOCTOR FROM RURAL PARAÍBA

The scientific quest to understand the power of Zika was moving deeper into the Northeast. In Campina Grande, Dr Adriana Melo works closely with Dr Melania Amorim, who is widely known in Brazil as an advocate of natural childbirth. Dr Melania studied medicine in Recife and now teaches in Campina Grande, where Dr Adriana was once her student. Both strive to advance humanized birth in the Northeast. Dr Melania's father, Prof. Joaquim Amorim Neto, was also an obstetrician, and the research institute coordinated by her and Dr Adriana is named after him. The two doctors also work with Dr Fabiana Melo, Dr Adriana's sister and a resident in obstetrics under Dr Melania; she was the one present at Géssica's delivery. These women are skilled in listening to their patients, soothing their pain and helping them focus on bringing their baby into the world.

By November 28, 2015, Pernambuco had registered 646 cases of microcephaly while Paraíba had tallied 248.[25] Statistics were similar for both states in terms of the proportion of total newborns. Nothing was being heard about the medical field in Paraíba; instead, the press was focusing on news and discoveries out of Recife, which was featured as the reference center.[26] Dr Adriana had a watchful eye on Dr Brito's comments on WhatsApp and was concerned about the hypothesis that the Zika virus causes microcephaly. Her own fetal medicine practice and the clinic at the university teaching hospital where she worked were brimming with women who had contracted the viral illness. Dr Adriana couldn't figure out why discoveries surrounding the Zika virus had jumped from mosquito to newborn. What about the pregnant women? Where were they?

Dr Adriana was performing 30 ultrasounds a day. Many expectant mothers were telling her stories about having caught a viral illness during pregnancy. If Zika was causing fetal microcephaly, as Dr Brito and Dr Vanessa claimed, why not back up a step and study the pregnant women? Dr Adriana wondered why her colleagues in Recife weren't asking this same question. It wasn't her pioneering spirit that pushed her to shift from clinician to great scientist but rather what her alert ears were capturing from patients and colleagues. Dr Fabiana, who is a big fan of her sister's, tried to persuade me that ever since she was little, Dr Adriana had nourished dreams of being a research scientist. "Look at this picture of her at the school science fair," Dr Fabiana said excitedly, grasping at an origin myth that her sister had never embraced.

Maria da Conceição Alcantara Oliveira Matias had been the first woman to attract Dr Adriana's attention. Conceição's ultrasound images were unusual; the calcifications were suggestive of infection but the brain abnormalities fit nothing that the doctor had learned in over 20 years of medicine. "She was in her 22nd week, and I couldn't understand the fetal brain," Dr Adriana said. "The cerebellum was very thin. I asked myself what the devil was going on." She met with two fellow specialists in fetal medicine, who were likewise surprised by the images; they had seen similar cases at a public maternity hospital. Conceição's first appointment was on September 29, 2015, and Dr Adriana spent October talking with her colleagues, driven especially by the buzz about microcephaly in Recife. Rumors were growing fast about the malformation and its possible ties with the Zika virus. In the days running up to the meeting of the Regional Board of Medicine chaired by Dr Brito, physicians in Pernambuco exchanged a flurry of messages on WhatsApp. Dr Adriana didn't know if they were completely true or interspersed with rumor.

Conceição's second appointment came on Friday, October 23. She'd spent a restless night and this time her husband Mário hadn't brought his camcorder. She was in tears when she arrived, the joy of her pregnancy now transformed into torment. She encountered a more serious Dr Adriana. "I've never seen this before," the doctor said, "but we're going to study it." The path would be to investigate what the ultrasound couldn't pick up, so the doctor ordered an MRI, plus an amniocentesis to check for chromosome disorders. Conceição said little that day. She and Mário had already decided to go to João Pessoa to get a second opinion from another specialist in fetal medicine. Conceição didn't tell Dr Adriana she was planning to consult with someone else; she couldn't say if she was embarrassed or just being protective of her privacy. The trip to João Pessoa wasn't her choice alone; she was also ceding to family pressure.

That night, Dr Adriana pored over the first technical report on microcephaly issued by the Pernambuco Department of Health. The document was officially released only on October 27, a sign of how much faster the news was spreading through alternative channels than the state bureaucratic network. "In the month of October 2015," the note said,

> the Executive Department of Health Surveillance was advised of the occurrence of 29 cases of microcephaly in children born since August of this year. . . . It is important to emphasize that, on the basis of available information, no relation can be drawn between this occurrence and any prior illness or malady. . . . This increase in [microcephaly] may be explained in various ways, including congenital infections (infections transmitted from mother to child during pregnancy) as well as other, non-infectious causes, especially in the first trimester of pregnancy.[27]

The report offered nothing new scientifically speaking, but as she scrutinized it, Dr Adriana kept remembering Conceição's tests. She turned to the medical literature but found no more than ten papers on the Zika virus, and the story was always the same: Uganda, Yap Island, French Polynesia.[28] She couldn't wait until Monday; she grabbed the phone and called Conceição to ask if she had experienced symptoms of Zika. When the woman confirmed that she'd had symptoms in her eighth week, Dr Adriana explained what was on her mind. Conceição still didn't mention her planned appointment in João Pessoa, which would be in a few days. She promised the doctor she too would read the state technical report and think things over.

Before venturing into the world of scientists herself, Dr Adriana decided to write Dr Kleber Luz:

We have been observing a rise in microcephaly rates here. In fetal medicine, we have observed hypoplasia of the *cerebellar vermis* and gross periventricular calcifications at roughly the 20th to 24th week of pregnancy, in addition to microcephaly. . . . I would like to know if the possibility of Zika has been investigated in the blood of newborns or the amniotic fluid of any fetus.

This was on November 4, 2015. Dr Kleber replied immediately: "This presentation is the same as the cases in Natal and Recife. If you can, send me your contact number." Just one week earlier, Dr Brito had nudged Dr Kleber into actively searching for women in Natal. Dr Adriana sent him her number and waited for his call, but it never came. She pressed him with another message: "Kleber, my question is whether or not the amniotic fluid of any of these fetuses has been studied, as we investigated cytomegalovirus, for example." For some reason, he never got back to her.

Conceição returned from her trip to João Pessoa and confessed to Dr Adriana that she had consulted with another specialist. She said the fellow had poked fun at the hypothesis raised by the doctor from rural Paraíba, but that she and Mário were interested in doing further research; the couple had read the state's technical report and decided they wanted to contribute to science. They were willing to donate amniotic fluid to see whether the Zika virus could be found hiding there. Out of curiosity, Dr Adriana asked why the specialist in João Pessoa had ridiculed her. Conceição, who is at home with medical jargon, said, "He told me it wasn't evidence-based science." Dr Adriana almost disputed this notion with the argument that "the first evidence is the observation of the specialist," but she let it go – after all, Conceição was in pain.

It was between Conceição's second appointment and the couple's decision to donate amniotic fluid that Géssica Eduardo dos Santos visited Dr Adriana's office, on November 6, 2015. Géssica's doctor in Juazeirinho had described the ultrasound images to her as "a little problem with the baby's head." He had also said she was accumulating amniotic fluid. Dr Adriana was struck by her new patient's images. "It was a very serious pattern," she explained to me, "and there were similarities with what I'd seen in Conceição. At that point, I thought Conceição's case might develop into Géssica's." Dr Adriana asked Géssica many questions, including whether she had contracted Zika during pregnancy. "Yes, in my fourth month," she replied. The obstetrician promised to get back to her with a diagnosis within a week.

Dr Adriana's call came earlier than expected. She asked Géssica to come in that same day if possible. The trip from Juazeirinho to Campina Grande takes an hour and Géssica would have to find a ride, so she could make it only the next day. Since it would be impossible to perform the procedure at a public health facility, the plan was to draw amniotic fluid in the doctor's private office and then send the sample to laboratory scientists in southern Brazil. On the afternoon of November 10, both Conceição and Géssica arrived in Dr Adriana's office in Campina Grande. It was the first time the two women met.

During amniocentesis, a thin needle is passed through the abdominal wall into the uterus and approximately 6 to 10 ml of amniotic fluid drawn out. The procedure is monitored by ultrasound to make sure neither the placenta nor the umbilical cord is affected. It was formerly thought that amniocentesis presents a risk to a pregnancy because it might trigger a miscarriage. While some risk exists, Dr Adriana has never seen any complications in her entire career as a doctor. Conceição and Géssica nonetheless had to sign an informed consent, which stated that the exam was to investigate the causes of suspected congenital infection.

To better view the images on the screen, Dr Adriana performs ultrasounds with the lights on low. That day she had further dimmed her office to create a more soothing atmosphere for the two women. Géssica went first. She told me she still remembers the burning sensation of the needle. The thin amniotic fluid rose slowly in the syringe, transparent as water. Dr Adriana asked herself what might be lurking in there. Géssica headed back to Juazeirinho right away, because the driver of the unregistered shuttle that was her precarious form of transportation was complaining about going back in the dark. Conceição was scared when her turn arrived; the needle seemed so big as it penetrated her belly. Besides, she had noticed Géssica's red eyes as she left the room. A cooler filled with ice packs awaited the tubes, which were to be sent off as fast as possible. Campina Grande didn't have an express postal service, so the cooler would have to go by plane. Conceição and Mário took the precious cargo to the airport, while Dr Adriana rushed off to a mass in honor of her only daughter's high school graduation.

The next day, the samples of Conceição's and Géssica's amniotic fluid reached Dr Ana Bispo, a researcher at Fiocruz in Rio de Janeiro. Dr Adriana had contacted Dr Bispo on November 5, between Conceição's second appointment and Géssica's first. Six days later, the material was at her lab in Rio. She ran the first tests and on the second day detected the presence of the Zika virus. Given the weight of this discovery, she knew her methodology might be questioned, so she contacted a colleague, Dr Renato Santana Aguiar, a virologist at Rio de Janeiro Federal University, and asked him to look into it further. "Do you suppose it's only Zika?" she asked when she handed him Conceição's and Géssica's samples.

A couple of days after drawing the amniotic fluid, Dr Adriana flew to São Paulo for a course on fetal neuroimaging. One of the instructors was a top expert in CMV, so Dr Adriana took the opportunity to discuss the two women's test results with him. The foreign physician was nonplussed by what he saw. He was sure it wasn't a CMV infection, but he said he'd like to repeat the tests. Dr Adriana says he asked her: "How can a country have hundreds of cases, and yet nobody has an answer?" On Friday, November 13, 2015, Dr Adriana called Conceição and Géssica with an urgent invitation. Could they leave immediately for São Paulo, expenses paid by the government? Eminent physicians were meeting in São Paulo, she explained, and the women would be seen by a foreign expert there.

The next day, the two couples met at the airport in João Pessoa for a frenzied weekend trip. Mário, the most seasoned traveler in the group, handled the tickets and explained the check-in and boarding process to Géssica and her husband Silvandro – it was their first time on a plane. When Géssica told me about the moment of take-off, her voice conveyed a mixture of excitement and apprehension. It was all so new. They arrived in São Paulo that same day. On Sunday, Conceição and Mário took advantage of the less hectic weekend traffic to stroll down Avenida Paulista, São Paulo's Fifth Avenue. They were amazed by the crowds. They stopped to pray at Imaculada Conceição Church, where they took their only photo on the trip. The women had their tests repeated that day as well.

Géssica grows sad when she remembers the doctor from abroad; she feels he was gruff with her, perhaps because he lacked the manner of a midwife from the Northeast, perhaps because of the language barrier. "It was a very painful moment. I was in anguish. The doctor explained how serious things were for my baby, the fact that my life was even at risk because I was accumulating a lot of amniotic fluid." Dr Adriana says she sensed Géssica's discomfort, but the doctor didn't show much concern for the woman's pain. In stark contrast with the usual behavior for many Brazilian doctors, he said nothing about hope, didn't react to her tears, and offered no comforting hug. Conceição's husband, who appeared oblivious to the doctor's cold demeanor, ventured a query: "Doctor, will my daughter feel my touch?" The doctor seemed put off by a question that might be deemed irrelevant in the context of matters of life and death. "I couldn't say," he replied.

It was Dr Adriana who stepped in to deliver the foreign doctor's verdict to Géssica and her husband. Like a doula, she knelt before the couple and asked them how much they wanted to know. "She crouched down between us, put her hands on my legs. She asked if we were ready. I always told her not to hide anything from me.

Whatever was happening, she had to be truthful," recalled Géssica. Dr Adriana translated the tragic diagnosis, the inviability of the fetus, and said it was up to Géssica and Silvandro to decide whether or not to terminate the pregnancy. Conceição's heart broke for Géssica, because she knew she herself would go back home certain her daughter would have a better chance than Géssica's baby; furthermore, as a physical therapist, she could make a difference in the child's life. But she knew Géssica would be saying farewell to her baby from that moment on.

Although unaware of it, Dr Bispo's research colleague, Renato Aguiar, was using the same metagenomic sequencing method that the Slovenian doctors had employed to detect the Zika virus in the body of Sofia's son Pietro. In different corners of the world, the expectant women were journeying along similar paths around the same time: Sofia donated Pietro's body to science on October 15; Conceição and Géssica donated amniotic fluid on November 10. With their own bodies, the two Brazilian women had proven the effects of Zika during pregnancy. Alone in Slovenia, without fanfare, Sofia had been one month ahead of them. A preprint of the article by Dr Jernej Mlakar and collaborators would be released one week before the publication of an article by Dr Adriana and her colleagues, in February 2016.[29] "Our group and the group from Slovenia found nothing but Zika," Aguiar told me. This confirmed the pathogen of the fetal sickness in molecular terms – Dr Brito and Dr Vanessa had already identified it clinically.

Shortly after disembarking in João Pessoa the following Monday, November 16, Dr Adriana called Dr Bispo, who informed her that the tests had been conclusive: the amniotic fluid contained ZIKV and no other virus. Neither said anything for a few moments as they processed the solemnity and the excitement of this finding. Then Dr Adriana immediately set about planning how to announce the discovery as quickly as possible, given the nature of the public health emergency. Her intrepid colleague, Dr Melania, was recovering from a bout of hemorrhagic dengue, which meant Dr Adriana would be on her own in dealing with any provocation from colleagues who did not consider her a scientist.

The obstetrician had no idea what the ramifications of her discovery would be. She was a female bedside physician from the poor, rural area of Paraíba now heading up a team of laboratory researchers. In a conversation between Dr Adriana, Dr Melania, and Dr Fabiana, I listened in as the three physicians pondered what might cause the greatest amazement: the fact that they were Northeasterners or the fact that they were women. Dr Melania was convinced their gender would matter more; Dr Adriana and Dr Fabiana contended it would be their accent. As they struggled to second-guess how Brazil's hierarchical scientific community would express its longstanding prejudices, I felt an urge to argue that the discussion was purely academic. As I saw it, whether they were viewed as females from the Northeast or Northeasterners who were females, the male scientists in the South would be astounded. But I refrained from fueling the debate.

Like Dr Gúbio Soares Campos, Dr Adriana made her first move by going to the press. She too understood her discovery as a spiritual mission. Although Dr Adriana often speaks with her patients in terms of Catholic saints and beliefs, she is a devout Spiritist. In her view, it wasn't just wisdom that made her ask about the amniotic fluid, much less any deep-seated desire to become a full-fledged scientist, contrary to her sister's origin myth. "It was spiritual illumination, for the good of humanity," she explained to me. Her of all people, a woman who chose fetal medicine because, in her own words, "I don't like death. I just want to celebrate life," found herself surrounded by forms and affidavits requesting authorization to terminate pregnancies because the accumulation of amniotic fluid was putting the lives of some of her Zika patients at risk.

After receiving confirmation from Dr Bispo, and even before leaving the airport in João Pessoa, Dr Adriana had called the biggest prime-time newscast in Paraíba and scheduled a live interview for that same night. Dr Adriana did not intend to tell anyone that Fiocruz had identified the virus in Conceição's and Géssica's amniotic fluid before the institute announced it. So why did she want to appear live on the most important television program in Paraíba? According to science protocols, hypotheses and results should only be commented on once they have been published in a journal. From this perspective, Dr Adriana's strategy was even more daring than Dr Gúbio's; when he made his press announcement about isolating the Zika virus, at least he was referring to blood samples at his own laboratory. "Look," Dr Adriana told me, "I was afraid people wouldn't want me to release the results, so I thought, I'll talk to the press today to say I drew [the fluid] and that we'd have the results by Wednesday, so there wouldn't be any type of pressure. I wanted to protect myself." Dr Adriana, like Dr Gúbio, felt somewhat intimidated by the scientific community in southern Brazil or by the workings of national public health policy. And to her chagrin, she wasn't misguided.

On her way to the television station, Dr Adriana stopped by the Paraíba Department of Health to notify them of the findings. A good number of doctors were there attending a meeting to discuss chronic diseases in the state. They paid no attention to her. She had to raise her voice, something out of tune with her mild manner. "Hey, folks, this isn't WhatsApp gossip," she insisted. The only person who thought her information merited attention was Dr Luzia Pinto, Campina Grande's health secretary. It seemed hard for the men present to accept the fact that a clinician had taken on the work of a scientist. For her part, Dr Adriana felt she had done her duty by notifying the state that she believed Zika was causing fetal microcephaly before she went to the press.

As Dr Adriana waited alone at the television studio that evening, she trembled with nervousness. The silence of the researchers in Recife continued to puzzle her. She wondered why it hadn't occurred to anyone else to do something as simple as draw amniotic fluid and check for the presence of the Zika virus; this would be routine when researching CMV. "Do you suppose the researchers in Recife all know but haven't said anything because Zika is such a serious matter?" she asked herself. Given these nagging doubts, she felt uneasy about declaring on television that she was investigating the hypothesis and that results would be released in a day or so.

Dr Adriana was on the air for nine minutes. The newscast presented a detailed report on the health care received by newborns with microcephaly in Paraíba, and physicians and experts shared what they knew about the epidemic. There was much talk about mosquitoes and how to eliminate their breeding grounds. Near the very end of Dr Adriana's interview, the newscaster asked: "Doctor, we've seen the Ministry of Health recommendations that mothers protect themselves against the *Aedes aegypti* mosquito. Does this in itself send a strong signal that the current microcephaly outbreak is caused by the mosquito?" Dr Adriana was evasive in her response but left plenty of hints about the upcoming announcement: "Well, in fact, we're converging more and more toward that hypothesis, but of course we can only be certain . . . once the virus has been detected in an affected patient. That's why it's so important for us to try to isolate it in the amniotic fluid."[30] Dr Adriana had accomplished what she set out to do: register her research on air.

Official announcement or not, the cat was out of the bag and the following days were tumultuous. Reporters from all over the world showed up at Dr Adriana's cramped office.[31] Conceição preferred to stay in the wings and refused to talk to the press, while Géssica became their spokeswoman, speaking time and again with Brazilian reporters and international correspondents. She let them take photographs of her, a pregnant woman with a big belly waiting for her day of mourning. Under the headline "'I still cry a lot', says woman in Paraíba expecting baby with microcephaly," one article featured a pair of photos that summed up Géssica's pain. In the first picture, she sits with her hands around her belly, rubbing her fingers together in uneasiness, a mother cradling her own body. She seems to look less at the photographer than into some far-off void. Over her shoulder we glimpse the Catholic saints and bible that adorn her home and her life. In the second picture, Géssica leans against the crib of the baby who will never come, mattress still wrapped in plastic. The only words she speaks during the interview are of pain: "Terribly sad." "It was really sad. I couldn't understand how serious it was. I kept asking myself why I have to go through this." "I still cry a lot because it upsets me so much."[32]

On November 18, 2015, Fiocruz published its own announcement of the discovery in an article on its website entitled: "IOC/Fiocruz detects presence of Zika virus in two cases of microcephaly" (in Portuguese).[33] There was no mention of Dr Adriana, only of "two pregnant women from Paraíba" and the state-of-the-art methodologies used by the laboratory. The same press release confirmed the identification of the genotype of the virus circulating in Brazil, that is, the Asian strain, which was sequenced by Dr Gúbio in April and Dr Cláudia in May 2015. The second chapter of the Zika epidemic in Brazil seemed to be coming to a close, but, to be on the safe side, Dr Cláudio Maierovitch, director of the Ministry of Health's Department of Communicable Disease Surveillance, opted for ambiguous language: "We cannot be categorical. But the presence of the virus is not merely a coincidence. . . . To date, there had been no evidence of a link between Zika virus and congenital malformation. For this reason, we are speaking in terms of a probable relation."[34] Just as Dr Adriana had resolved to limit her comments on air to the fact that research was underway, perhaps the Ministry of Health had likewise opted to keep quiet about its own upcoming announcement.

Dr Adriana understood science. She knew her two cases might not offer enough evidence to warrant confirmation of a causal relation between the Zika virus and microcephaly. When she failed to receive the honors due a scientist who has made a major discovery, she resigned herself to the ways of science – especially because this wasn't what she was truly after. She would wait for control studies using a greater number of samples than just Conceição's and Géssica's before she would use the term "causality" with the patients in her office.

There were other reasons no one was rushing to affirm that Zika causes microcephaly. The last time the women of the world had felt a similar public health impact was during the terrifying rubella epidemics of the early 1960s,[35] which left thousands of babies with congenital rubella syndrome, first identified in the 1940s. The risk that a fetus will suffer damage if the mother catches rubella during the first ten weeks of her pregnancy is as high as 90 percent, a rate that falls after the 18th week.[36] When an epidemic hit Europe in 1962 and then another struck the United States in 1963–1964, there was as yet no vaccine, which was only developed in the late 1960s.[37] On November 28, 2015, Dr Adriana was surprised by this headline: "Ministry of Health confirms relation between microcephaly and Zika virus."[38] The confirmation was based not on her work but on a single identification by the Evandro Chagas Institute in Belém, and the discoverer was identified as the director of the institute, Dr Pedro Vasconcelos, the man who had been urged by Dr Celso Tavares to use Zika primers to investigate the Currais Novos samples nearly one year earlier.

The Ministry of Health issued a solemn press release:

This Saturday, the Ministry of Health confirmed the relation between the Zika virus and the microcephaly outbreak in the Northeast region. The Evandro Chagas Institute, a ministry agency in Belém, Pará, submitted the results of tests conducted on a baby born in Ceará with microcephaly and other congenital malformations. The presence of the Zika virus was detected in blood and tissue samples. Based on this finding from the baby, who passed away, the Ministry of Health deems as confirmed the relation between the virus and the occurrence of microcephaly. This is an unprecedented situation in worldwide scientific research.[39]

Given that the results of Dr Adriana's research had been announced ten days earlier, at this point the only "unprecedented" aspect of the situation was that a prestigious Brazilian research institute was now confirming her findings.

According to the Evandro Chagas Institute, "the baby presented microcephaly and other congenital malformations."[40] The infant in question was a girl who survived for five minutes after birth; there is no mention of the altruistic woman who donated her daughter to science.[41] Nor is there any mention of the bedside physicians who told the mother about their suspicions, who broached her about the matter of donating her child for research purposes, or who may even have been the ones to send the corpse or organs to the laboratory in Belém.

In the official history of the epidemic, the discovery of the causal relationship between the Zika virus and microcephaly was not made by Dr Adriana in rural Paraíba but by the Evandro Chagas Institute, a reference laboratory attached to both Fiocruz and the Ministry of Health. Vasconcelos explained in an interview at the Evandro Chagas Institute press office:

> The case of this baby enabled us to factually link irrefutable laboratory data with the causal relationship between microcephaly and Zika virus. In this context, one case suffices to prove the relation because: the latter was suspected clinically, there was a temporal association with increased cases of microcephaly during the Zika epidemic, and, further, Fiocruz detected the virus in the amniotic fluid of two pregnant women whose fetuses had been diagnosed with microcephaly.[42]

Vasconcelos is an eminent virologist at the institute and the fact that the discovery came from there lent greater clout to the Ministry of Health's request that WHO classify the microcephaly epidemic as a Public Health Emergency of International Concern, a request that was lodged on November 29, 2015. The Brazilian press heralded Vasconcelos as the discoverer of causality: "'Our hands and feet are tied,' physician says about Zika. Pedro Fernando da Costa Vasconcelos, researcher at the Evandro Chagas Institute in Pará, has proven the relation between the virus and microcephaly."[43]

The news saddened Dr Adriana. She didn't need a science manual to understand that two cases are more than one, or that Conceição's and Géssica's amniotic fluid had already proven what the institute proclaimed as news. Her unhappiness was much less because she was being unfairly disregarded and more because the announcement had implications for her ambitions as a scientist in the epicenter of the epidemic: with the country's main research centers assuming the starring role, research funds would be unequally distributed.

On December 1, 2015, PAHO released its first Epidemiological Alert on the neurological syndrome, congenital malformations, and Zika virus infection. It was the PAHO/WHO system's first official announcement concerning the implications for public health in the Americas. The document mentions the detection of ZIKV in the amniotic fluid of "two pregnant women from Paraíba," but the highlighted discovery is the one by the Evandro Chagas Institute: "The Brazil Ministry of Health established the relationship between the increase in occurrence of microcephaly and Zika virus infection through the detection of Zika virus genome in the blood and tissue samples of a baby from the state of Pará."[44] The newborn from Ceará had vanished from history.[45]

Dr Adriana's melancholy was short-lived. As a bedside physician, she believed her patients' pain took precedence over her own feelings about not being recognized. Not long after Fiocruz confirmed that ZIKV crosses the placenta, a new worry struck her. Some women were concealing their itching and red rashes during pregnancy. Like their fellow neuropediatricians in Recife, Dr Adriana, Dr Melania, and Dr Fabiana had set up a clinic for microcephaly cases, where the patients were pregnant women at risk for Zika. Open every Friday, it quickly became the unofficial reference clinic for microcephaly in rural Paraíba, where mothers-to-be came to hear their sentences handed down. The quiet hallway that served as a waiting room was always crammed with pregnant women, often in the company of their mothers, not often accompanied by men. Dr Adriana described it as a place of great suffering.

Nothing could be done to fix the calcifications or microcephaly; moreover, the diagnosis was pronounced when the gestation was already advanced, or – as Dr Melania put it – "when the women are already very pregnant." Abortion is common among women of reproductive age in Brazil, but the procedure is illegal and therefore clandestine, and it is usually performed in the first weeks of gestation.[46] Only if her life is at risk can a woman request special authorization to terminate her pregnancy. Fetal malformations were being diagnosed roughly between the 20th and 24th weeks, by which time a woman had effectively gained the status of mother-to-be in the eyes of society. To escape a sentence that offers no remedy and no choice, some women started lying when Dr Adriana asked if they had experienced symptoms during pregnancy. "Did you have symptoms of Zika?" "No, I didn't."[47] If the obstetrician noticed the woman casting her eyes downward or lowering her voice, she would press on: "Because I only see Zika patients here, so why did they send you to me?" The answer was always the same: "Because I had dengue. It wasn't Zika." Dr Adriana skirted the frightening issue of Zika during pregnancy and listened to their stories of dengue unfold, reading Zika between the lines all the while. In her mind, if she had insisted that the rash had been caused by Zika, not dengue, she would have lost her patient's trust right from their first meeting. These women had found a way to resist: they attached a label to their viral illness that would have a less dramatic impact on their lives. Dengue wouldn't touch the fetus; Zika would leave its footprints on the brain.[48] While listening to the conversations between Dr Adriana and the women in the ultrasound room, I wondered about the epidemiological surveys then underway. When women were asked if they had had a rash, itchiness, or Zika during pregnancy, what were they telling science?

If world science took time to affirm causality, Dr Adriana never had any doubts.[49] For her, as for many other researchers, the uncertainty was whether congenital Zika syndrome is triggered by the Zika virus alone or if other, prior illnesses or other viruses circulating in Brazil might not also play a role. The day after the announcement that ZIKV had been found in Conceição's and Géssica's amniotic fluid, Dr Adriana was back at her office – which she actually never left, even after her 15 minutes of fame as a research celebrity. The truth of the matter was that she had arrived at the discovery precisely because she has always been a bedside physician. If she was also a researcher now, she still never failed to remind the world what she had said on television back when the news about causality was still a veiled secret:

These results are not mine. These results belong to Guilherme's mother; these results belong to Catarina's mother. We must remember they are not just numbers. There are parents behind these children; there are families behind them. These children have names; these children have life; and these results in truth belong to these mothers.[50]

# PATIENT ZERO

Brazil's "patient zero," the twin whose brother was not affected by Zika, lives in Custódia, a small town in Pernambuco, 340 kilometers from Recife, the capital. His father, Paulo Joaquim Peterson Pereira, is a geography teacher and also owns a small shop. He takes good care of his children and wife, a young woman who doesn't want their sons exposed or the details of their lives made public. It was her husband, an articulate speaker, who had identified himself to the press as P.J. For the purposes of this book, the couple agreed I could interview Paulo; he would be his family's spokesperson and only his name would appear.

Their son was affected by Zika during the first month of gestation, back when the women of the Northeast thought they were just fighting an allergy, bug, or, like Paulo's wife, possibly mild dengue. The family wants their privacy respected not out of shame, but because talking about their sorrow over the birth of a son with a small head isn't paramount right now. What matters most to them is shouting about their son's needs today; Paulo wants his voice to serve as a manifesto for life. The twin is being well cared for; the family has turned the words "early stimulation" into both a form of affection and a political gesture. The wife quit her job for the time being and stays home so she can stimulate their son to the maximum during his early development.

One day during her pregnancy, the wife had felt her skin burning; the next day she was over it. She never mentioned the episode of brief discomfort to her doctor during her prenatal visits, because she didn't even think of it as being sick; it was one of those bad days a woman has to put up with when she's pregnant. She'd been taught that being a mother, as the saying goes in Brazil, means "suffering in paradise." The couple's first two children would arrive together and their trials and tribulations would be doubled too. The pregnancy had been "planned, programmed, and wanted" – the string of adjectives is uttered by Paulo, who has mastered the skill of talking about his son's microcephaly with utmost thoughtfulness. If there is anything tragic about their situation, it is not the existence of their son but the fact that an epidemic gave him the name "patient zero" and then assigned him to oblivion.

Paulo doesn't want the story of his son or his family to be one of pain or lamentation. If he was once intent upon discovering what had affected the boy, now he seeks to answer another question: "Why have we been isolated?" While the label "patient zero" bothers him, he still realizes that theirs is a position of relative privilege: "Right here in Custódia, there are kids with microcephaly who are several months older than my son." The twins turned one in July 2016. Paulo understands that the term "patient zero" is less about their son being the first fetus affected by Zika during pregnancy but more about his being the first patient who awakened medicine to vertical transmission, for history is not told from the perspective of those in pain but by those who possess the voices to tell it. Patient zero was the title bestowed by science; he was the first child whose microcephaly prodded Dr Vanessa Van der Linden to take notice.

Paulo repeats the question to me: "Why have we been isolated?" The epidemic has been forgotten. At the time of our interview, in June 2016, Brazil continued to talk about its political crisis and the arrests and imprisonment of powerful people charged with corruption. And the woman in Custódia who had a baby with microcephaly before patient zero was even born never went to Recife to report her case. This woman is anonymous; she doesn't feel isolated like Paulo's family, because a poor, rural laborer like her never expects any recognition, not even for being alive. Patient zero's family doesn't want to talk anymore about the painful ultrasounds, about their repeated prenatal visits where nothing was explained to them, about the wife's perpetual struggle as she carried two babies in her belly without knowing what to make of the calcifications on the brain of one of them.

Paulo and his wife managed to survive the initial lack of definition on the part of science. "The doctors didn't know what was going on," he said. If he remains in distress, it's because he thinks the doctors still don't know what's going on. "Do you suppose something might eventually happen with the other twin?" Paulo asks me. It is a question without an answer. Shortly after giving birth, his wife moved to Recife with the newborns because there was a huge Zika outbreak in Custódia. People flooded doctors' offices and urgent care, and the family didn't know if the virus would attack their children. If there is a sharp edge to Paulo's voice when he complains about their isolation, it is especially because he wonders whether something is lurking silently inside the other twin. "We know so little about this disease," he observes in dread.

The couple understands that there is something else about their son's status as patient zero: they stand on one of the top rungs of the socioeconomic ladder in their corner of the Northeast, like Maria da Conceição Alcantara Oliveira Matias in rural Paraíba, the first woman who Dr Adriana Melo identified as carrying a baby damaged by Zika. Both families went to private healthcare providers and could afford to repeat tests and allow medicine to investigate what science didn't yet know. Paulo asked questions similar to those asked by Sofia Tezza, the Italian woman who had written Dr Kleber Luz even before a causal relationship had been established between the Zika virus and microcephaly. All of these women and men transformed themselves into scientists when the epidemic struck them deep at home, and hope spurred their resistance.

Paulo shared almost nothing of his family's story with the press. Quite to the contrary, he was upset by the "twins' overexposure on TV and in the papers," exposure that neither he nor his wife had authorized. In any case, what he wanted to say about his own life was not what reporters wanted to know. He granted three interviews and in all three implored: "I want our identities to remain confidential." He felt duped by those who broke their pledge to protect his privacy and he has refused to speak to the press since. He only agreed to talk to me because Dr Vanessa assured him that he could read the story prior to publication.

"Now," Paulo told me, "it's time to resist. The Brazilian government has to answer this question: Why have we been isolated?" He's not talking about geographic isolation. The family owns a car and several times a week makes the 160-kilometer trip for rehab in the neighboring town, where the twin receives early stimulation. Nor is this isolation an intellectual matter. Paulo has made himself a student of medicine; he talks about tests and risks like an expert in the Zika virus, neurology, and rehabilitation.

Before and after patient zero, there were dozens of other children in Custódia and other towns in the Northeast. "There are many, many women who are alone with their children, who have microcephaly. Many babies are dying; others need to be hospitalized," Paulo says, lending the notion of isolation further nuances. His children made it through the first year after the epidemic. Their family altruistically contributed to scientific research by donating blood, test results, and medical histories. One year later, they were continuing their struggle to find out what science had discovered about their children, because the researchers never gave them the results of the tests done on the twin. Paulo is troubled by this. "What do they know that I don't?"

"I served research, I served the government. I want my rights respected." And his voice rises in pitch to claim what is owed him. He quickly goes on to supplement his political discourse with a request for understanding: "It does me good to express myself; it helps me find meaning in all this." In one of the few press interviews he granted, the reader can sense him getting upset: "Gosh, if I'd known, I would have done something." I ask him what he thinks he could have done for his son. His illusion is that he could have saved him; he has a fantasy about going back to the past and spending the pregnancy somewhere far from Pernambuco. I imagine Paulo and his wife fleeing to a place outside their lives, escaping the mosquitoes and the isolation that have beset them.

There was nothing patient zero's family could have done. Brazil has grappled with copious mosquitoes for 40 years. *Aedes aegypti* was there before Zika arrived. Paulo grows bewildered when he speaks of the Northeast. He asks himself whether the Zika virus really exists, or if the problem might not actually be something else – after all, "why just in the Northeast?" When he posed the question, I didn't know how to respond, except by offering the formal explanations of science. But in truth, I do know the answer. It happened here, in the Northeast, because it is this land of slavery, of masters and captives, that has made Brazil one of the most unequal countries in the world.

# THE AFTERMATH

Northeast Brazil was the epicenter of the country's epidemic of congenital Zika syndrome (which many in this region continue to call simply "microcephaly"), and the Northeastern states that reported the highest concentration of babies affected by the malady were Pernambuco and Paraíba. The first epidemiological report issued by the Brazilian Ministry of Health indicated that 739 cases of microcephaly had been reported nationwide by November 21, 2015; the report did not enter into the merit of how many cases had been confirmed or discarded.[1] The ministry's seventh epidemiological report, released on January 2, 2016, put the total at 3,174 cases; by the release of report number 32, issued nearly six months later, the figure had reached 8,165.[2]

Behind these figures were women and newborns. Newborns' heads were measured right after birth and if the circumference was smaller than the benchmark for that month, the infant was immediately reported. The next step was to investigate the case and either confirm or dismiss it. During the investigation, the mother had to take her baby back and forth to tests and appointments. Paraíba and Pernambuco have few centers of medical investigation; in any case, the timeline for medical diagnosis moves more slowly than the timeline for women who are waiting for science to provide answers. For a mother, what matters most is knowing test results as soon as possible so she can begin proper care.

Paulo Pereira, patient zero's father, knows of mothers in his hometown of Custódia who failed to notify any public health agency of their children's microcephaly, children who were in fact born before his son and who were already a year old at the original writing of this book, but who belong to a category not to be found in Brazil's epidemiological surveillance system: *ignored cases*. What is even more disquieting is that recent studies have suggested that some newborns affected by the Zika virus have a normal head circumference at birth.[3] And then there are the sick women and children who can be categorized as ignored because healthcare policies offer them no means of recovery.

For every newborn who is reported, a full-time caregiver must be available to take the infant to medical appointments and, if congenital Zika syndrome is diagnosed, to early stimulation therapy as well. In Northeast Brazil, family life centers around children, and their care is entrusted to women, so the caregiver will quite likely be the child's mother or grandmother or, in large families, perhaps an aunt, older sister, or cousin. If none of these are available, it may even be a neighbor who takes the child to his appointments. A broad network of women moves into action to help the mother whose child has been reported, investigated, confirmed, or even ignored. I heard no stories of this task being outsourced to nannies or daycare. In rural communities and among the poor, an epidemic is experienced differently than it is by women from Brazil's urban elites.

I spent many days at the microcephaly clinic at Pedro I Hospital in Campina Grande, one of the country's first centers specialized in the early stimulation of babies with congenital Zika syndrome. Caregivers generally had to make two trips a week for 30-minute sessions. Their journeys are long and transportation, precarious; saddest to say, the public at large sees the latter as a perk handed out to the families by local government. Transportation costs are covered for only the infant plus one caregiver, but as the child grows, carrying him gets harder. And for many of these women, staying at home rather than returning to their jobs represents another onus.

Cristiana Alves da Silva, a single mother who lives on a modest farmstead in Monteiro, a small town in Paraíba, is one of the women I met. Cristiana makes a five-hour round trip to take her son, Davi Luiz, to early stimulation. Before her pregnancy, she worked as a sharecropper. In June 2016, she was awaiting approval of social benefits to help care for her child, who demands full-time mothering. A foreign photojournalist captured Cristiana just as she lives: sitting alone inside a humble home, her son in her arms, light from a dim bulb above seeping into the pitch black yard outside.[4] Cristiana was just one of the women in her town who endured the turbulent passage through the world's largest outbreak of Zika. She became pregnant with Davi Luiz precisely in December 2014.

At the clinic in Campina Grande, I met some of the few fathers who are also caregivers. Maybe there were more fathers hidden inside their homes, but I rarely saw them make back-and-forth trips with their children for medical appointments. Joselito Alves dos Santos was one who did. Married to Maria Carolina Silva Flor and father to Maria Gabriela, he always attended meetings and had an active presence on social media. Like Paulo, patient zero's father, he talked about rights in the aftermath of a public health crisis that had injured his child.[5] I cannot affirm that men abandoned their homes and families after their children were born with congenital Zika syndrome, but this was a hot topic in the press and on social media in Brazil in the months following the epidemic.[6]

Social media and apps, especially WhatsApp, played a central role in the exchange of information, hypotheses, and rumors.[7] Even as this book was being translated into English, in early 2017, I was following dozens of chats a day between mothers who had formed WhatsApp groups. In those conversations, I never read any tales of men running off, but this may simply be because no one in the Northeast expects them to take care of children. On the other hand, there were many stories of men who were weary of listening to their baby's nonstop crying and of couples who grew frustrated by the demands of caregiving and the virtual absence of government support. Family poverty and endless pilgrimages to hospitals were the most common topics among the women who, like the doctors in "CHIKV, the mission," relied on WhatsApp to exchange information and better cope with what the epidemic left in its wake.

Dr Fabiana Melo had used WhatsApp to introduce Géssica Eduardo dos Santos to Alessandra de Sousa Amorim. The doctor knew Géssica was waiting to pass João Guilherme's baby things on. Alessandra's son Samuel had just been born with congenital Zika syndrome. Her husband is a mason's laborer; the couple and their four children survive on a family income below the poverty line. Alessandra forwarded me the text messages she exchanged with Géssica:

"I'm Géssica, from Juazeirinho. You know what happened. It hurts, but it's in God's hands, God is in charge. . . . God has prepared a beautiful gift for you."

"I have faith."

"And how's Samuel?"

"He's fine. I have faith that God will give you a perfect baby, just like you've dreamed of."

"I'm going to bring you some things for Samuel."

"I'm going to take a picture of Samuel to show you."

"I'm going to bring you the things as a present for him."

"You're going to give them away? Don't you plan on having another baby?"

"I don't plan on having any kids right now. I want to get over this loss."

"I'm sorry I asked, honey. Don't get mad at me."

"It's natural for people to ask. I don't get mad."

"We'll see each other tomorrow, God willing. I'd like to hold Samuel in my arms. It'll be my first contact with a child with microcephaly."

"You won't notice Samuel's head very much. You can hold him."[8]

Stories like Gessica's and Alexandra's have been commonplace in the groups of mothers I follow, where conversations alternate between displays of overmothering and bouts of despair about how to meet their children's needs. Together these women learn how to deal with everyday discrimination; they have been stalwart advocates of their right to bare their children's heads in public, undisguised by any cap or hat. And they grieve the lack of a cure or treatment for microcephaly. They grow excited when a headline announces an advance in stem-cell research or when they hear that a faith healer has performed a miracle. They protect each other, challenge physicians and diagnoses, and exchange information on new manifestations of congenital Zika syndrome. It was through this exchange of messages that many discovered that some of the children have trouble swallowing. Other women received advice about the importance of demanding an expert medical report to guarantee access to certain forms of social assistance.

The figures on the microcephaly epidemic shocked Brazil at first. In late 2015, some authorities and the press took comfort in announcing that the epidemic was on the wane, though there was no way of knowing whether the drop in numbers was attributable to new parameters for reporting head circumference, the seasonal nature of mosquito infestations (the months of greatest risk may be March to May),[9] or the shifting prevalence of one virus over the other in this triple epidemic (2016 ended up being the year of chikungunya).[10] In the southern hemisphere, the truth of the matter is that the medical world will only have a measure of the impact on subsequent generations of women and children struck by Zika at the close of each calendar year, since the peak risk of mosquito bites comes in the early months. From 2014 to 2015, there was a 2,023 percent increase in reports of newborns with microcephaly in Brazil.[11] From January to June 2016, reported cases rose 157 percent. Almost all of these babies lived in the Northeast. A study by Giovanny França shows that 97 percent of definitive or probable cases of congenital Zika syndrome originated in states that account for 28 percent of all births in Brazil.[12]

The history of the first year of Brazil's Zika epidemic saw two consecutive feats of science: the discovery that the virus was circulating in the country and the discovery of congenital Zika syndrome. The key players were bedside physicians, laboratory scientists, and, above all, the women who caught "mild dengue" and ended up caring for babies born with congenital Zika syndrome, regardless of whether their case fell into the category of reported, confirmed, or ignored. In devising public health policies during the epidemic, Brazil talked more about mosquitoes than people. The slogan of the public health campaign was "A mosquito is not stronger than an entire nation."[13] In telling the history of these discoveries and the disputes over recognition, this book has gone back to the lives of the women and children, which is what should be of paramount importance during a public health emergency of global proportions.

In all of this, the approach to doing science and announcing discoveries was quite Brazilian. Perhaps this Brazilian approach is actually the "correct way" to address public health emergencies in countries on the periphery of global science. The research was done by bedside physicians; the results were released to the press before they were published in scientific journals; doctors and patients told the story together.[14] It is safe to say that it wasn't only their concern with the common good that inspired physicians and scientists to go to the press before communicating with their peers; theirs was also a concern with their potential access to Brazil's unequally distributed research funding. After all, the ones who blazed trails during this epidemic were physicians and scientists from the Northeast, and they were eager to make their voices heard and receive due recognition.

These individuals also sought to protect themselves, for while there was much solidarity between those in the Northeast and their colleagues in southern Brazil, there were also contests to see who could publish a groundbreaking discovery or announce a major accomplishment first, a phenomenon typical of science everywhere.

Moreover, while Northeasterners were active in discovering that the Zika virus was circulating in Brazil and in the hypothesis of vertical transmission, the traditional authorities of Brazilian science, concentrated in the South, soon took over as spokespersons in the pages of international publications. This immediate replication of the reigning social stratification within Brazilian science should come as no surprise, because a single event cannot in itself be expected to undermine unequal patterns of resource distribution.

Just a little over three months passed from Dr Vanessa Van der Linden's identification of patient zero in her office to the day the Brazilian Ministry of Health declared a public health emergency. Some lauded the government for its speed in responding to signs of the microcephaly epidemic. But credit for the swiftness of this response must go first and foremost to doctors and researchers on the periphery of Brazilian science rather than to any government policy. Furthermore, this speedy response came in tandem with muddled statements and fits of silence on the part of the government. In December 2015, then Health Minister Marcelo Castro slipped back into old ways of promoting women's health when he declared: "Sex is for amateurs; pregnancy is for professionals."[15] Regrettably, the minister's lapse wasn't the only such blunder committed in Latin America when the Zika epidemic swept the region. Governments in countries like El Salvador called for women to avoid pregnancy until 2018.[16] No public health policy can consider abstinence from either sex or conception to be reasonable recommendations for controlling an epidemic that has multiple forms of transmission, in this case both by vector and through sex.

If, on the one hand, this neo-Malthusian approach to reproductive health policies showed a lack of respect toward thousands of women, on the other, it clearly signaled the direction the Brazilian government preferred to take in addressing the consequences of the epidemic: it made the mosquito vector the villain. This is not to deny that *Aedes aegypti* must be eliminated as rapidly as possible but, given the overwhelming lack of family planning resources and support in Brazil, this line of attack is far from a magic bullet. The joy of pregnancy vanished from Brazil's Northeast with the news of Zika congenital syndrome, and Dr Adriana Melo was not overstating things when she described the corridor extending from her waiting room to the ultrasound room as "death row" and her office as the place where the women hear their sentence handed down.

In these pages, I chose not to explore recent research on transgenic mosquitoes,[17] mosquitoes purposely infected with bacteria,[18] mosquitoes sterilized by gamma or X-rays,[19] or larva-killing biolarvicides,[20] teas, or oils.[21] If these new weapons prove successful, the mosquito may vanish or be rendered incapable of transmitting the disease. Any of these options would offer a spectacular solution to the epidemic, and the mosquito would no longer be the perfidious emblem of the Brazilian family. But until such time as these discoveries materialize, and until a vaccine reaches the market, the Zika virus demands immediate, serious responses, above all because it presents a special risk for women of reproductive age and their future babies. We cannot speak of people in terms of ageless, sexless masses; it is young women who are pregnant, or planning to be, who are now terrified by the mere act of living in the land of Zika. Simply because they are poor Northeasterners, ordinary women have been ignored by policies that should respond to suffering in a country as unequal as Brazil's.

Should the epidemic find its way into urban areas, women from the elites will find alternative ways to ensure a safe pregnancy despite Zika.

If neither the confirmation of the Zika virus in Brazil nor even the discovery of congenital Zika syndrome constituted a scientific revolution, representing instead normal science, what is indeed extraordinary about Brazil's epidemic is the state of abandonment to which thousands of women were relegated after their children's cases were reported, investigated, confirmed, or ignored. A third chapter is waiting to be added to the story of Zika in Brazil, a chapter in which addressing women's reproductive health needs becomes tantamount to addressing public health needs.[22]

The discovery of the vertical transmission of the Zika virus has shown us that protecting reproductive health depends on guaranteeing rights, including access to contraceptive methods and the right to a safe abortion. It is disturbing to think that only a global threat might force Brazil to look inside itself and recognize that the urgent need for care and protection is not limited to getting rid of a mosquito but includes looking after the women and children affected by the Zika virus or at risk.

# IMPLICATIONS FOR WOMEN WORLDWIDE

"The Committee advised that the recent cluster of microcephaly cases and other neurological disorders reported in Brazil, following a similar cluster in French Polynesia in 2014, constitutes a Public Health Emergency of International Concern (PHEIC)."[1] On the evening of February 1, 2016, following a nearly four-hour-long meeting with members of the International Health Regulations Emergency Committee on Zika virus, Dr Margaret Chan, then WHO Director-General, declared the fourth global health alert in history.[2] PHEICs had been previously declared in 2009 for swine flu[3] and in 2014 for polio[4] and Ebola.[5] WHO had been strongly criticized for its slow response to Ebola.[6]

The epidemic demanded an efficient response. By the time WHO declared the PHEIC, indications were strong that Zika could be transmitted vertically.[7] Studies likewise indicated that transmission could occur sexually,[8] by blood transfusion,[9] or through urine and saliva.[10] Furthermore, the Zika virus had been detected in breast milk.[11] The warning issued by WHO left it clear: it was not Zika itself, even in epidemic form, that had warranted the alert; the real global threat was the risk that a pregnant woman might pass the virus on to her fetus, bequeathing her child congenital Zika syndrome. Two months later, on April 7, 2016, WHO released a statement confirming the hypothesis: "Based on a growing body of preliminary research, there is scientific consensus that Zika virus is a cause of microcephaly and Guillain-Barré syndrome."[12] While much remains to be learned about how the virus works, the identification of causation was decisive to the shaping of health policy and international research agendas.[13]

Between February 2016, when Dr Chan made the initial announcement, and April 2016, when WHO declared that the virus causes congenital Zika syndrome, a vast body of research was published. The scientific community was working hard to understand the events in Brazil and get ahead of the global threat of further dissemination of the virus. The term "threat" was not the hype of journalists playing on people's fears; it signaled the very real power of a virus that can be transmitted a number of ways.[14] And for the countries where *Aedes aegypti* circulates – more than 100 by 2015 – the biggest and most immediate menace was the vector behind Brazil's Zika epidemic.[15] By February 2, 2017, Zika itself had been reported in 76 countries and territories; in 59 of those, it had been detected for the first time after 2015.[16] By that same month, the only places in Latin America where autochthonous transmission had not occurred were Chile and Uruguay[17] (though Uruguay had seen cases of Zika illness brought in by travelers).[18] In other words, the virus had penetrated the borders of all other countries in Latin America.

Figures on vertical transmission and increased cases of GBS were expected to parallel those of Brazil. By February 2017, Colombia, Dominican Republic, El Salvador, French Guiana,

French Polynesia, Guadeloupe, Guatemala, Honduras, Jamaica, Martinique, Puerto Rico, Suriname, and Venezuela – like Brazil – had reported a surge in cases of GBS,[19] while newborns with congenital Zika syndrome virus had been reported in 28 countries and territories besides Brazil. In most cases, the sickness had spread through autochthonous transmission; in a few, it had been carried by pregnant travelers, as in Slovenia (Sofia Tezza, the Italian who had lived in Rio Grande do Norte, Brazil, during her early pregnancy), Spain (women who had traveled to Colombia and Venezuela), and the United States (possibly women who had visited Brazil, Guatemala, or Belize). There was as yet no information on Canadian cases.[20]

The epidemic was raging and science was making haste, but vital questions remained unanswered: What lineage was circulating in the countries that had detected Zika? What were the implications of the virus's return to Africa, via Cape Verde, now in the form of the Asian lineage?[21] Was there a risk of vertical transmission and congenital Zika syndrome in every country where the virus had recently landed? At the onset of the epidemic, Colombia – which shares a border with Brazil – set up a broad-reaching system to monitor the effects of the virus, but its numbers remain unclear.[22] The figures in Colombia may prove lower than Brazil's not only for environmental reasons, such as rate of mosquito circulation or type of climate, but also because Colombian law permits a woman to terminate her pregnancy if it presents a risk to her health.[23] Right after it had been proven that the congenital syndrome was linked to the Zika virus, Colombia's vice-minister of health, Fernando Gomez, was asked whether Brazil should follow his country's example and reform its laws. He replied: "I can't voice an opinion about another country, but I can say that it is an important choice for a woman. . . . One of the most frequent justifications for terminating [a pregnancy] here is the risk of mental suffering for the woman."[24]

Colombia had quickly recognized the need to adopt integral measures to protect women's reproductive health. Dr Ana Cristina González-Vélez, former national director of public health with Colombia's Ministry of Health and Social Protection, compared Brazilian and Colombian policies with these words: "Unlike Brazil, Colombia's protocol stresses the importance of information in the following terms: 'pregnant women with Zika virus infection should be informed of the existence of an association between the infection and congenital anomalies of the newborn's cranium and central nervous system'."[25] Colombia released its protocol in February 2016, immediately following Dr Chan's announcement.

It is challenging to conduct studies on the public health impact of the various forms of Zika virus transmission, especially when the mosquito vector is circulating in the country or an epidemic is already underway. Firm evidence of sexual transmission of Zika illness has thus been limited.[26] By February 2017, 13 countries had reported sexual transmission based on individual case studies of men who had traveled to countries in Latin America and returned to their homes (Germany, Argentina, Canada, Chile, Peru, Spain, United States, France, Italy, New Zealand, Portugal, United Kingdom, and Netherlands).[27] In many of these countries, it was possible to test for sexual transmission of the Zika virus precisely because the mosquito vector was absent.

On June 14, 2016, the WHO Emergency Committee on Zika virus released the following statement:

The Committee concluded that there is a very low risk of further international spread of Zika virus as a result of the Olympic and Paralympic Games as Brazil will be hosting the Games during the Brazilian winter when the intensity of autochthonous transmission of arboviruses, such as dengue and Zika viruses, will be minimal and is intensifying vector-control measures in and around the venues for the Games which should further reduce the risk of transmission.[28]

In the same statement, the committee reiterated WHO's earlier recommendations that pregnant women not travel to countries where the Zika virus circulates and that, following their visit to Brazil, their sexual partners should abstain from sex during pregnancy.

WHO also recommended that athletes and visitors to the Brazilian Olympics choose air-conditioned accommodation where doors and windows were kept closed to keep mosquitoes from entering; follow the travel advice provided by their countries' health authorities; consult a healthcare provider before traveling; use insect repellents and wear clothing that covers the body; and avoid cities and areas with no piped water or poor sanitation.[29] In short, WHO advised that it was safe to travel to Brazil during the epidemic, as long as the traveler stayed in an air-conditioned hotel and wore clothing to minimize skin exposure. What was most troublesome, however, was that WHO insisted sexual abstinence could be taken seriously as a method for protecting health and an alternative to the use of barrier methods like condoms.

In the history of epidemics caused by sexual transmission, abstinence policies have proven inefficacious for at least two reasons: (a) no studies have ever been done on the actual behavior of those purportedly practicing abstinence; (b) for people who are sexually active, abstinence recommendations are hard to comply with.[30] Countries seeking to expand forms of protection for women of reproductive age must diversify long-term family planning methods to include options like IUDs and hormone injections or barrier methods like condoms. But the most problematic issue in calling for abstinence as an alternative to the condom is the lack of clarity regarding what to abstain from. Coitus alone? Oral sex as well? Zika can be sexually transmitted because the virus is found in semen and one case of transmission via oral sex has been reported.[31] According to the Centers for Disease Control and Prevention (CDC), a person who has Zika can pass the virus to his or her sex partner during vaginal, anal, or oral sex without a condom or through the sharing of sex toys.[32] It is not yet known whether women infected with the Zika virus can transmit the disease sexually to their male or female partners.[33]

In Brazil, researchers at the University of São Paulo (USP) who specialize in mathematic modeling announced that the risk of a traveler acquiring Zika in Brazil during the 2016 Olympic or Paralympic Games and then carrying the illness back home was almost nil, approximately three cases per 100,000 visitors. "Roughly 15 people would be infected," the article stated, "with 10 asymptomatic and 5 symptomatic cases."[34] Since these scientists felt the threat to global health was so low, they decided to poke fun at those who asked for the sporting event to be postponed: "If you aren't pregnant and decide to skip the Olympic Games in Rio de Janeiro because you're afraid of catching Zika, you can look for a better reason. There are many others."[35] In July 2016, the state of Rio de Janeiro had the highest number of confirmed cases of congenital Zika syndrome outside the Northeast. The figure had leapt from two confirmed cases in February, when WHO declared its global alert, to 87 cases by July 9.[36] Additionally, Rio was the state with the most cases of Zika virus infection in the country, with 43,516 notified cases.[37]

But what the USP researchers' mathematical model does not show is the complexity of Zika transmission. When the male partner of a pregnant woman travels to a country infested by Zika and then returns sick to his homeland, he can infect his partner, who may in turn pass the virus to her fetus. When the Brazilian mathematicians did their risk calculations, they failed to take into account the actual probability of sexual transmission to a pregnant woman and subsequent vertical transmission, because science does not even possess this information. CDC guidelines for June 2016 recommended that pregnant women with partners who had traveled to an area with Zika should practice safe sex or abstain from sexual activity for at least six months upon their return.[38]

Science still has much to learn about Zika. The risks of sexual transmission and later vertical transmission top the list of worrisome uncertainties, given their impact on the lives of women of reproductive age. Moreover, if, as international analysts have insisted, there is indeed the threat of a worldwide Zika epidemic, this threat is not equally distributed among nationalities, genders, or age brackets. Herein lies the true threat: as Zika continues its march across the globe, pregnancy will become a time of anguish for all women of the world, as it is now for the women of Northeast Brazil.

# NOTES

## TELLING THE STORY

1 Congenital Zika syndrome is the more accurate term for the adverse effects of Zika, which include a group of signs and symptoms of which microcephaly is but one feature (BRITO, 2015; CHAN et al., 2016; COSTA et al., 2016; MIRANDA-FILHO et al., 2016). However, most Brazilian women and even the World Health Organization (WHO) continue to use the term "*microcephaly.*"

2 DINIZ, *Zika*, 2016.

3 Transcribed from an exchange of messages within a WhatsApp group.

4 BRAGA; VALLE, 2007.

5 MLAKAR et al., 2016.

6 MELO et al., 2016.

7 In February 2016, "acute Zika virus disease" was added to Brazil's list of diseases and public health events subject to mandatory reporting; included was a special line item for cases involving pregnant women (BRASIL. Ministério da Saúde, 2016a). According to Administrative Ruling no. 104, of January 25, 2011, in turn based on International Health Regulations 2005 (IHR 2005): "A Public Health Emergency of National Concern . . . is an event that presents the risk of spreading disease to more than one state . . . which requires the prioritization of diseases and other public health events subject to immediate reporting, regardless of nature or origin, subsequent to a risk assessment, and which may require an immediate nationwide response" (BRASIL. Ministério da Saúde, 2011). On December 8, 2015, a form was released for reporting public health events related to microcephaly and/or changes to the central nervous system. See http://bvsms.saude.gov.br/bvs/saudelegis/

gm/2011/prt0104_25_01_2011.html. Prior to the epidemic, WHO head-circumference-for-age charts were used for this purpose.

8 VICTORA et al., 2016.

9 ARAÚJO et al., 2016.

10 GRENS, 2016; CASOS . . ., 2016. In epidemiology, causality has to do with the conditions, events, and pathogenic agents that trigger a disease. A spurious correlation is a correlation without verified causality, that is, where two phenomena occur together but are not linked.

11 REINACH, 2016a, 2016b, 2016c.

12 BRASIL não registrava . . ., 2016. Specificity and sensitivity are important concepts in epidemiology and have been at the center of controversies over the microcephaly epidemic in Brazil. Specificity refers to the precision of a measurement while sensitivity has to do with the detection of true positives. At the outset of the epidemic, in November 2015, a head circumference of 33 cm was considered normal for newborns, meaning that any newborn presenting a smaller circumference should be reported as suspected microcephaly. Those concerned with greater accuracy argued that reducing the cutoff for normal head circumference would stem excessive reporting, while those concerned with greater sensitivity held that the cutoff should not be changed because, if an error were to occur, it would be better to overreport newborns at potential risk than to delay treatment of actual bearers of the neurological syndrome. The arguments favoring greater precision won out, and the cutoff for head circumference in reporting microcephaly underwent a series of changes in Brazil (VICTORA et al., 2016).

13 LATIN AMERICAN COLLABORATIVE STUDY OF CONGENITAL MALFORMA-TIONS, 2015.

14 BRASIL. Ministério da Saúde, 2015a. Implemented in the 1990s, Brazil's Live Birth Information System (SINASC) registers congenital anomalies in newborns. It was only after the Zika epidemic triggered a spike in reported microcephaly cases that the Ministry of Health created an online form called the Public Health Event Report Form: Microcephaly. Guidelines were made available through Brazil's Surveillance and Response Protocol for Zika, the first version of which was released on December 7, 2015 (BRASIL. Ministério da Saúde. Secretaria de Vigilância em Saúde, 2015).

15  Drawing inspiration from Thomas Kuhn's classic *The Structure of Scientific Revolutions*, I use the term "extraordinary event" to mean one that subverts established scientific practice, or "normal science." In Kuhn's own words: "'Normal science' means research firmly based upon one or more past scientific achievements, achievements that some particular scientific community acknowledges for a time as supplying the foundation for its further practice" (KUHN, 2012, p. 10).

16  YUKI; HARTUNG, 2012.

17  Arbovirus is the ecological term used to refer to viruses that are transmitted by arthropods (insects and arachnids, for example) as a way of completing their life cycles.

18  HAYES, 2009.

19  DINIZ, 2016.

20  DUFFY et al., 2009.

21  GUILLAIN; BARRÉ; STROHL, 1916. The disease was named after Jean-Alexandre Barré and George Charles Guillain, the doctors who identified it.

22  DICK, 1952.

23  PubMed holds more than 25 million open-access references to biomedical and life sciences articles; it is run by the National Center for Biotechnology Information (NCBI) in the United States.

24  The world's chief academic journals in the field of medicine agreed to enforce two practices to hasten dissemination of information on the epidemic: rapid peer review and open-access publication. This was consonant with the understanding that public health emergencies demand data sharing, an agreement reached in September 2015 by WHO and key biomedical journals, including *The British Medical Journal, Nature Journals, The New England Journal of Medicine*, and the seven PLoS journals (WORLD HEALTH ORGANIZATION, 2015). Yet even with this open door policy toward science communication, two things in Brazil prompted findings to be released first through the press and only months later through science media: the language barrier and the fact that the doctors involved were viewed first as clinicians and only secondarily as researchers.

25  PAN AMERICAN HEALTH ORGANIZATION, 2016a.

26  WORLD HEALTH ORGANIZATION, 2016e. WHO is responsible for declaring Public Health Emergencies of International Concern. When a country identifies a potential global threat, it has 24 hours to report

the focal point to WHO. On November 11, 2015, Brazil's Ministry of Health declared a national emergency; on November 29, it advised WHO of the potential global emergency. On December 1, PAHO issued an epidemiological alert, but another two months would lapse before Dr Margaret Chan, then WHO Director-General, declared an international emergency.

27  SENRA, 2016.
28  PAN AMERICAN HEALTH ORGANIZATION, 2016c.
29  PAN AMERICAN HEALTH ORGANIZATION, 2016c, p. 5.

## POSITIVE FOR ZIKA

1  Va'a outrigger canoe racing originated in Polynesia. Two thousand athletes from 18 countries took part in the event in Rio de Janeiro, held in Rodrigo de Freitas Lagoon.

2  A phylogenetic lineage is a group of organisms sharing certain morphological and physiological similarities and displaying differences vis-à-vis other lineages of the same species.

3  FAYE et al., 2014.

4  Australia, South Korea, Iran, and Japan were the only Asian teams to play in the World Cup in Brazil (in accordance with FIFA's classification of Asian).

5  FARIA et al., 2016, p. 347.

6  FARIA et al., 2016, p. 347.

7  WHO SCIENTIFIC GROUP, 1985.

8  CENTERS FOR DISEASE CONTROL AND PREVENTION, n.d.; GUBLER, 2002.

9  LOPES; NOZAWA; LINHARES, 2014.

10  CASSEB et al., 2013.

11  ZANLUCA; SANTOS, 2016.

12  CASSEB et al., 2013.

13  The same group of researchers conducted similar studies on mice, rabbits, and guinea pigs (DICK, 1952).

14  These data are from the WHO "Zika situation report" for February 2, 2017, which does not specify the lineage of the virus circulating in each country (WORLD HEALTH ORGANIZATION, 2017). The fact that 59 countries reported circulation of the Zika virus following 2015 may

at it belonged to the Asian family, which had been detected
̶.̶a̶z̶i̶i̶, but there is no reliable way to confirm this.

15  DICK; KITCHEN; HADDOW, 1952; DICK, 1952.

16  Lyle R. Petersen and collaborators state that 13 cases have been
described in the medical literature (PETERSEN et al., 2016); Mark Duffy
and collaborators affirm that there have been 14 (DUFFY et al., 2009).
These numbers are negligible for a disease with epidemic potential.

17  GRARD et al., 2014.

18  DUFFY et al., 2009.

19  DURAND et al., 2005; SAVAGE et al., 1998.

20  LANCIOTTI et al., 2008.

21  JOUANNIC et al., 2016.

22  CAO-LORMEAU et al., 2016; IOOS et al., 2014. According to WHO,
Guillain-Barré syndrome is a rare condition in which a person's immune
system attacks the peripheral nerves; it can affect people of any age but
is more common among adults and males. Most people recover fully,
even from the most severe cases (WORLD HEALTH ORGANIZATION,
2016b).

23  CAO-LORMEAU et al., 2016; CAUCHEMEZ et al., 2016. French Polynesia
and Brazil issued epidemiological alerts on the possible connection
between Zika and microcephaly at practically the same time. French
Polynesia's epidemiological surveillance report for epidemiological
week 48 of 2015 (November 23–29) addresses the matter under the
title "Congenital cerebral malformations possibly linked to Zika
virus" (in French). Eighteen cases of brain malformations had been
reported following the Asian country's Zika epidemic in 2014, and the
document states: "Investigations are looking into all possible exposures
but the hypothesis of ZIKV infection appears to be the most likely."
On November 24, 2015, French Polynesia notified WHO about an
increase in cases of fetal malformation (POLYNÉSIE FRANÇAISE, 2015).

24  VOGEL, 2016a.

25  BRASIL. Ministério da Saúde. Secretaria de Vigilância em Saúde, 2014.
In September 2014, the Ministry of Health issued its first official report
on the autochthonous transmission of chikungunya, but the news
media had been reporting sicknesses caused by the virus since July of
that year, for example, in Rio de Janeiro (DOIS . . ., 2014).

26  BRAGA; VALLE, 2007.

27 FULLERTON; DICKIN; SCHUSTER-WALLACE, 2014.

28 HONÓRIO et al., 2015; TEIXEIRA et al., 2015.

29 LENHARO, 2014.

30 JOFFÉ, 1986.

31 BECKER, 2016.

32 SANTOS, 2015, p. 19.

33 PETERSEN et al., 2016.

34 INSTITUTO EVANDRO CHAGAS, n.d.

35 RODRIGUES, 2015.

36 MANSON, 2014, p. 159.

37 The investigatory techniques employed in Brazil were conventional methods consonant with recognized technological science. RT-PCR, or reverse transcription polymerase chain reaction, allows researchers to amplify trace amounts of DNA millions of times and thus detect the presence of a specific virus or set of viruses (CAMPOS; BANDEIRA; SARDI, 2015; FARIA et al., 2016; ZANLUCA et al., 2015).

38 The first primers used by Dr Cláudia Duarte dos Santos were generic for flavivirus, which was the same research method used by the Evandro Chagas Institute. During her second round of testing, the virologist used ZIKV-specific DNA sequencing primers. Her research identified the genome circulating in Brazil as Asian.

39 ZANLUCA et al., 2015.

40 DOENÇA . . ., 2015.

41 MELO, 2015.

42 KNIPE; HOWLEY, 2001.

43 CAMPOS et al., 2016.

44 Dr Antônio was attending the European Congress of Clinical Microbiology and Infectious Diseases (ECCMID).

45 Aliança refers to Aliança Hospital in Salvador, the private facility where Dr Antônio was working in January 2015. All samples in which the Zika virus was identified in fact came from Camaçari.

46 IDENTIFICADO . . ., 2015. The discovery went virtually unnoticed on the world stage. The international press only assigned the topic to its ongoing news cycle once a relation had been drawn between the Zika virus and fetal microcephaly.

47 BALM et al., 2012; CAMPOS et al., 2015.

48 CIENTISTAS . . ., 2016.

49 GERMANO, 2015.

50 COSTA JUNIOR, 2015.

51 TV NBR, 2015. Chioro erred in his numbers. The Evandro Chagas Institute confirmed four samples from Camaçari as positive. Although the laboratory in Bahia had identified the Zika virus in eight, only seven were validated pursuant to identification criteria.

52 BAHIA, 2015.

53 WORLD HEALTH ORGANIZATION, 2015.

54 ZANLUCA et al., 2015.

55 The journal *Emerging Infectious Diseases* used the expression "first detection" for the last time in the title of a paper released in 2002. Seemingly synonymous terms like "discovery" and "novel," which are not strictly the same scientifically speaking, still appear.

## THE FIRST GENERATION OF WOMEN

1 Press reports often misidentified Sofia Tezza as a "Slovenian woman."

2 MLAKAR et al., 2016.

3 COGHLAN, 2016; VOGEL, 2016b.

4 FORMENTI, 2015a; LEITE, 2015.

5 MICROCEFALIA . . ., 2015.

6 EXAMES . . ., 2015.

7 In the documentary *Zika*, I tell the story of five women from the Cariri region of Paraíba. The movie closes with Géssica's story (DINIZ, *Zika*, 2016).

8 MELO et al., 2016.

9 These are their real names. I interviewed most of them, filmed some, and spent a great deal of time with others during physical therapy sessions at Pedro I Hospital in Campina Grande, Paraíba. I followed them all on a daily basis through the WhatsApp mothers group, where a steady stream of messages has been sent back and forth since February 2016.

## FOOTPRINTS OF THE VIRUS

1 COELHO, 2015.

2 FRANCO, 2015.

3 GUILLAIN; BARRÉ; STROHL, 1916.

4 YUKI; HARTUNG, 2012.

5 YUKI; HARTUNG, 2012.

6 OEHLER et al., 2014.

7 IOOS et al., 2014, p. 306.

8 FRANK; FABER; STARK, 2016.

9 BONITA; BEAGLEHOLE; KJELLSTROM, 2010.

10 PAN AMERICAN HEALTH ORGANIZATION, 2015.

11 PERNAMBUCO. Secretaria de Saúde. Secretaria Executiva de Vigilância em Saúde, 2015a.

12 PERNAMBUCO. Secretaria de Saúde. Secretaria Executiva de Vigilância em Saúde, 2015b.

13 COSTA, 2015.

14 PERNAMBUCO. Secretaria de Saúde. Secretaria Executiva de Vigilância em Saúde, 2015a.

15 On November 11, 2015, the state of Pernambuco released a clinical and epidemiological protocol for microcephaly; the document stated that cases of "microcephaly smaller or equal to 29 cm at birth" had prompted the alert about a "microcephaly epidemic" (PERNAMBUCO. Secretaria de Saúde. Secretaria Executiva de Vigilância em Saúde, 2015c).

16 Prior to the epidemic, Brazil had no specific metric for recording microcephaly, but a head circumference of 33 cm was considered normal. On December 8, 2015, in its protocol for Zika-related microcephaly, the Ministry of Health reduced head size from 33 cm to 32 cm (BRASIL. Ministério de Saúde, 2015b). On January 21, 2016, PAHO suggested 31.6 cm for girls and 32 cm for boys (PAN AMERICAN HEALTH ORGANIZATION, 2016b). On March 10, 2016, in a protocol pertaining to microcephaly and/or changes to the central nervous system, the Ministry of Health made another change, this time reducing the measurements to 31.5 cm for girls and 31.9 cm for boys (BRASIL. Ministério de Saúde, 2016b). In other words, a head size that was deemed small in October 2015, at the outset of the epidemic, was no longer considered small in March 2016. These reductions in the cutoffs for reporting microcephaly totaled 1.5 cm for girls and 1.1 cm for boys.

17 The same day that Sofia Tezza wrote to Dr Kleber, she posted a comment on the Brazilian science blog Divulga Ciência, which had reported on Dr Cláudia Duarte's paper about the Zika virus, in a

commentary entitled "First description of Zika virus transmitted in the country warns of spread of the disease" (in Portuguese). Sofia apparently copied her email to Dr Kleber right into her online comment. On November 18, the news blog replied: "Dear Sofia, I don't know if you've been following the recent cases of a large number of babies who are being born in Pernambuco with microcephaly. The main hypothesis is precisely that the mothers were infected by Zika virus during pregnancy, which simply reinforces what happened to you" (BARATA, 2015).

18  Recent studies have shown that some mothers of newborns presenting congenital Zika syndrome probably had Zika during pregnancy although they had presented no apparent symptoms, like a rash or itchy skin (FRANÇA et al., 2016).

19  Karyotype, a profile of a person's chromosomes, is used in diagnosing genetic disorders.

20  LEITE, 2015.

21  CREMEPE . . ., 2015.

22  BRITO, 2015; MIRANDA-FILHO et al., 2016. There are in fact cases of newborns diagnosed with congenital Zika syndrome whose head circumference is within the so-called normal range; in other words, they do not display microcephaly as a sign of the syndrome.

23  A portion of the work done during this period was later published (ARAGAO et al., 2016).

24  COSTA, 2015.

25  BRASIL. Ministério da Saúde, 2015c.

26  The earliest news out of Paraíba dates from the first half of November 2015; there was a tone of relief since cases there were much fewer than in Pernambuco. "Pernambuco is facing an emergency situation and Paraíba also has cases of microcephaly" read the headline on one news site (PE tem situação . . ., 2015). The authorities quoted in the reports were from outside Paraíba, including Dr Brito, Dr Kleber, and the Ministry of Health.

27  PERNAMBUCO. Secretaria Estadual de Saúde. Secretaria Executiva de Vigilância em Saúde, 2015d.

28  Mark Duffy's study on the outbreak of Zika on Yap Island made no mention of Zika virus infection among pregnant women. At that time, nothing was known about the incidence of Zika virus among

mothers-to-be or about the symptoms of the disease during pregnancy. In the earliest studies based on clinical data in Brazil, the figures on rates of ZIKV among pregnant women differed sharply from what was expected. Furthermore, data on vertical transmission during the second world outbreak, in French Polynesia, were being released in parallel with data on the epidemic in Brazil (DUFFY et al., 2009).

29 CALVET et al., 2016; MLAKAR et al., 2016. It is worth noting that on January 5, 2016, before either the Slovenian or Brazilian teams had published their papers, Dr Adriana Melo and collaborators published a physician alert in the journal *Ultrasound in Obstetrics & Gynecology*, in which they reported on the two cases and the presence of ZIKV in amniotic fluid. This is considered the first official medical publication on the vertical transmission of the Zika virus (MELO et al., 2016).

30 JORNAL DA CORREIO, 2015.

31 Dr Adriana Suely de Oliveira Melo is cited as a source in nearly 1,000 of the references that I surveyed, all published since she began researching Zika.

32 XAVIER, 2015.

33 IOC/FIOCRUZ, 2015.

34 FORMENTI, 2015c.

35 LÖWY, 2016a, 2016b.

36 In regards to Zika, research on the risk of a pregnant woman transmitting the disease to her fetus is still incipient. Early in the epidemic, Dr Laura Rodrigues, a Brazilian researcher at the London School of Hygiene and Tropical Medicine, moved to Recife. She has published more on Zika than any other scientist worldwide. Rodrigues has observed large variations in risk estimates, from 1 percent to 29 percent. "As expected," she writes, "the estimates are different, but are they consistent with a single underlying risk or, alternatively, will risk be dependent on other factors, such as the presence of clinical symptoms or previous dengue infection?" (RODRIGUES, 2016a, p. 2071).

37 PLOTKIN, 2006.

38 MINISTÉRIO . . ., 2015.

39 BRASIL. Ministério da Saúde. 2015a.

40 MINISTÉRIO . . ., 2015.

41 This information on the newborn's brief life is found in the Ministry of Health's protocol on microcephaly and changes to the central nervous

system (BRASIL. Ministério da Saúde. Secretaria de Vigilância em Saúde, 2016a).

42 INSTITUTO EVANDRO CHAGAS, 2015. In a report dated December 18, 2015, the Evandro Chagas Institute mentions three cases of death caused by ZIKV: an adult male in Maranhão, a teenage girl in Pará, and the baby girl in Ceará, who lived only five minutes. However, when the Ministry of Health announced the causal relationship on November 28, 2015, the institute mentioned only the baby girl.

43 AZEVEDO, 2015.

44 PAN AMERICAN HEALTH ORGANIZATION, 2015.

45 The PAHO document errs in describing the baby girl from Ceará as a case from Pará.

46 By age 40, one in five women in Brazil has had at least one abortion (DINIZ; MEDEIROS, 2010). These are ordinary women, many of whom already have children; most take drugs to abort.

47 The reference study on attack rates – that is, the number of people hit by a new virus within a given population – and on the rate of people with Zika illness presenting symptoms was quickly lifted from Yap Island and applied to Brazil, yielding the prediction that only one in five people would present symptoms (DUFFY et al., 2009). The population of Yap Island was 7,391 at the time of the Zika outbreak, whereas Pernambuco had a population of over 9 million at the time of the Brazilian epidemic, with 1.5 million residing in Recife alone. In number of inhabitants, Yap Island is more like Ingazeira, the smallest municipality in Pernambuco. The study by Mark Duffy was transposed to Brazil as if it were a collection of absolute truths about how Zika behaves in epidemic form. The attack rate on Yap Island was estimated at 14.6 per thousand inhabitants while the rate for cases presenting symptoms was estimated to be about 20 percent. No one has any idea of these numbers in Brazil.

48 A recent study by Giovanny França and collaborators analyzed data from 1,501 newborns who were classified as suspected cases of congenital Zika syndrome. Of total cases, França arrived at a predictive value of 71.1 percent for rash during pregnancy linked to subsequent neurological damage to the fetus. Knowing which symptoms may predict the syndrome is important to defining policies for reporting and investigating cases of an epidemic. The authors suggest that

Brazilian guidelines concerning the centrality of reported rashes during pregnancy may need to be revisited. Symptoms may not be evident, either because a woman has only mild Zika, which goes unreported, or because many women simply do not seek medical attention (FRANÇA et al., 2016). Furthermore, Dr Adriana's insight suggests that something else may be going on as well: women may be denying symptoms evocative of Zika. This means epidemiologists must ask culturally adept questions if they are to arrive at a proper diagnosis of infants with the syndrome.

49 WHO only announced a "scientific consensus" that Zika can cause microcephaly and GBS in April 2016 (WORLD HEALTH ORGANIZATION, 2016a).

50 JORNAL DA CORREIO, 2015.

# THE AFTERMATH

1 The following week, the state of Paraíba scored highest in the concentration of reported newborns (BRASIL. Ministério da Saúde. Centro de Operações de Emergências em Saúde Pública sobre Microcefalias, 2015a).

2 BRASIL. Ministério da Saúde. Centro de Operações de Emergências em Saúde Pública sobre Microcefalias, 2016a.

3 FRANÇA et al., 2016.

4 GOODMAN; SAVARESE, 2016.

5 DINIZ; BRITO, 2016.

6 RESK, 2016.

7 There were two sets of apparently baseless rumors about what was causing the microcephaly epidemic, neither of which led to any serious research agendas. The first was a controversy over the possible involvement of the MMR or rubella vaccines; the second concerned larvicides. Studies were recently published on the relation between the yellow fever vaccine and the microcephaly epidemic, but as of July 2016, these were still exploratory (CAVALCANTI et al., 2016).

8 This conversation was transcribed verbatim from the women's WhatsApp messages.

9 Given the continental size of Brazil as well as the impacts of climate change, the notion that there is a risk of infection only during peak

months has met with harsh criticism; it may be more accurate to consider the entire year (FULLERTON; DICKIN; SCHUSTER-WALLACE, 2014).

10  Dr Celso described the treatments that clinicians devised for the chikungunya outbreak that followed the triple epidemic in the Northeast. In his words, these treatments had something of "supernatural, irrational science" about them, even though they were prescribed by medical doctors: "Meloxicam 7.5 mg + Tramadol 40 mg + Cimetidine 200 mg + Hydrochlorothiazide 25 mg. 1 tablet at bedtime." In the eyes of a good doctor, this prescription borders on sorcery, since it mixes an anti-inflammatory used to treat arthritis, an analgesic, a drug for stomach pain, and a diuretic, which is generally used to control blood pressure.

11  The percentage increase from 2014 to 2015 was calculated using figures from the Brazilian Ministry of Health (BRASIL. Ministério da Saúde, 2015b; BRASIL. Ministério da Saúde, 2015c).

12  "Definitive cases" are those in which the Zika virus was actually detected in the newborn; probable cases are those diagnosed through imaging (FRANÇA et al., 2016).

13  BRASIL. Ministério da Saúde, 2016c.

14  In using the term "correct way," I do not mean to dispute the fundamental importance of peer-to-peer communication in promoting science. My observation pertains to the context of the epidemic and the fact that the Brazilian Northeast is very much on the periphery of science.

15  FORMENTI, 2015b.

16  DALTON, 2016.

17  ESTUDO . . ., 2016; CANCIAN, 2016.

18  BACTÉRIA . . ., 2016.

19  AGÊNCIA, 2016; VILLELA, 2016.

20  BORGES, 2016.

21  COSTA, 2016; RODRIGUES, 2016b.

22  There is little indication that the third chapter of the Zika epidemic will place women at the center of political concerns. In the realm of morality, an unexpected but most welcome step forward was taken when Pope Francis stated that "avoiding pregnancy is not an absolute evil" (POPE, 2016). Furthermore, speaking in reference to the risk that

the Zika epidemic presented to women of reproductive age in Brazil, the pope qualified as acceptable the use of artificial contraception, in addition to so-called natural methods.

## IMPLICATIONS FOR WOMEN WORLDWIDE

1 WORLD HEALTH ORGANIZATION, 2016e. Dr Pedro Fernando da Costa Vasconcelos, of the Evandro Chagas Institute, is the only Brazilian member of the WHO Emergency Committee. The paper by Lavínia Schuler-Faccini and collaborators, released on January 29, 2016 in *Morbidity and Mortality Weekly Report*, a publication of the Centers for Disease Control and Prevention, is considered the key study behind the WHO announcement. In it, Schuler-Faccini analyzed data from 35 newborns with microcephaly (SCHULER-FACCINI et al., 2016).

2 WORLD HEALTH ORGANIZATION, 2016e.

3 WORLD HEALTH ORGANIZATION, 2009.

4 WORLD HEALTH ORGANIZATION, 2014a.

5 WORLD HEALTH ORGANIZATION, 2014b.

6 HAYDEN, 2016.

7 CALVET et al., 2016; FRANÇA et al., 2016; MELO et al., 2016; MLAKAR et al., 2016; RASMUSSEN et al., 2016; SCHULER-FACCINI et al., 2016. On November 18, 2016, WHO issued a statement that "Zika virus and associated consequences remain a significant enduring public health challenge requiring intense action but no longer represent a PHEIC as defined under the IHR" (WORLD HEALTH ORGANIZATION, 2016g).

8 ATKINSON et al., 2016; D'ORTENZIO et al., 2016; DECKARD et al., 2016; FOY et al., 2011; TURMEL et al., 2016; MANSUY et al., 2016; MUSSO et al., 2015b.

9 MARANO et al., 2016; MUSSO et al., 2014.

10 MUSSO et al., 2015a.

11 BESNARD et al., 2014; DUPONT-ROUZEYROL et al., 2016.

12 WORLD HEALTH ORGANIZATION, 2016a.

13 Two fundamental questions are whether the virus acts alone or in combination with other pathogens or whether its teratogenic effect depends on a woman's prior medical history – for example, on whether she has dengue antibodies in her blood.

14 The fear that this epidemic would spread well beyond the borders of

Brazil gradually crept into the pages of the international press, but the notion that it was a serious threat to the world only took firm hold closer to the Olympic Games in Rio de Janeiro (BAJAJ, 2016; SALZBERG, 2016; GRAIL, 2016; BUCCI, 2016; PREIDT, 2016; WILLETS, 2016; ASSAM, 2016; SANTORA, 2016; SINGER, 2016; EL ZIKA . . ., 2016).

15 As of 2015, the *Aedes aegypti* mosquito circulated in over 100 countries and *Aedes albopictus* in more than 80 (KRAEMER et al., 2015).

16 WORLD HEALTH ORGANIZATION, 2017.

17 CENTERS FOR DISEASE CONTROL AND PREVENTION, 2016b.

18 URUGUAI . . ., 2016.

19 WORLD HEALTH ORGANIZATION, 2017.

20 WORLD HEALTH ORGANIZATION, 2017.

21 On May 20, 2016, the Institut Pasteur in Dakar announced the sequencing of the Zika virus then circulating in Cape Verde; it was the same Asian lineage as the one in Brazil, from where it perhaps came. The WHO Regional Director for Africa voiced apprehension about this discovery: "The findings are of concern because it is further proof that the outbreak is spreading beyond South America and is on the doorstep of Africa." By May 8, 2016, more than 8,000 suspected cases of Zika had been reported in Cape Verde along with three cases of congenital syndrome (WORLD HEALTH ORGANIZATION, 2016b). One of the current hypotheses is that the Asian lineage is linked to vertical transmission to fetuses, while the African lineage is not (ZHU et al., 2016).

22 GIL, 2016. In 2016, a study by researchers from Colombia's National Institute of Health was following 1,850 pregnant women infected by the Zika virus. Through April 2016, four children in the group presented the congenital syndrome while further cases were under investigation (PACHECO et al., 2016). To obtain a true measure of risk among pregnant women, the number of women who terminated their gestation after contracting Zika illness would also have to be known.

23 Colombia's restrictions on abortion were among the most stringent in Latin America, but in 2006 its Constitutional Court authorized abortion under the following circumstances: risk to a woman's health or life; serious malformation of the fetus incompatible with survival; rape; and use of reproductive technologies without a woman's consent (COLOMBIA, 2006).

24 FORMENTI, 2016.

25 GONZÁLEZ-VÉLEZ, 2016.

26 MCNEIL JR, 2016.

27 WORLD HEALTH ORGANIZATION, 2017.

28 WORLD HEALTH ORGANIZATION, 2016d.

29 WORLD HEALTH ORGANIZATION, 2016f. In the first version of the document, released on May 12, 2016, WHO also suggested that tourists refrain from visiting poor or heavily populated areas in Brazil.

30 DAILARD, 2003.

31 WORLD HEALTH ORGANIZATION, 2016c.

32 CENTERS FOR DISEASE CONTROL AND PREVENTION, 2016c.

33 WORLD HEALTH ORGANIZATION, 2016c.

34 In a letter published in *The Lancet*, the authors stated that the risk of infection among tourists in Brazil was 3 to 59 cases (MASSAD, 2016).

35 TOLEDO, 2016.

36 BRASIL. Ministério da Saúde. Centro de Operações de Emergências em Saúde Pública sobre Microcefalias, 2016b.

37 BRASIL. Ministério da Saúde. Secretaria de Vigilância em Saúde, 2016b.

38 CENTERS FOR DISEASE CONTROL AND PREVENTION, 2016a; WORLD HEALTH ORGANIZATION, 2016c.

# BIBLIOGRAPHY

## BOOKS

BONITA, R.; R. Beaglehole; and T. Kjellstrom. *Epidemiologia básica*. 2nd ed. São Paulo: Santos, 2010, http://apps.who.int/iris/bitstream/10665/43541/5/9788572888394_por.pdf (accessed July 4, 2016).

KNIPE, David M.; P.M. Howley, eds. *Fields Virology*. 4th ed. Philadelphia, PA: Lippincott Williams & Wilkins, 2001.

FULLERTON, Laura M.; S.K. Dickin; and C.J. Schuster-Wallace. *Mapping Global Vulnerability to Dengue Using the Water Associated Disease Index.* Hamilton, ON: United Nations University, 2014.

KUHN, Thomas S. *A estrutura das revoluções científicas.* 5th ed. São Paulo: Perspectiva, 1998.

KUHN, Thomas S. *The Structure of Scientific Revolutions.* 50th anniversary ed. Chicago, IL: University of Chicago Press, 2012.

MANSON, Patrick. *Manson's Tropical Diseases*, ed. J. Farrar, P.J. Hotez, T. Junghanns, G. Kang, D. Lalloo, and N. White, 23rd ed. Saunders Elsevier, 2014.

SANTOS, Milton. *Por uma outra globalização: do pensamento único à consciência universal.* 15th ed. Rio de Janeiro: Record, 2015.

## FILMS

DINIZ, Debora. *Zika.* São Paulo: Itinerante Filmes, 2016, www.youtube.com/watch?v=j9tqtojaoGo (accessed February 22, 2017).

JOFFÉ, Roland. *The Mission.* Produced by Fernando Ghia and David Puttnam. United Kingdom: Warner Bros, 1986.

## SCIENCE JOURNAL ARTICLES

ARAGAO, M. de F. Vasco; V. Van der Linden; A. Mertens Brainer-Lima; R. Ramos Coeli; M.A. Rocha; P. Sobral da Silva; and M.D. Costa Gomes de Carvalho et al. Clinical features and neuroimaging (CT and MRI) findings in presumed Zika virus related congenital infection and microcephaly: retrospective case series study. *The BMJ*, pp. 1–10, 2016, www.bmj.com/lookup/doi/10.1136/bmj.i1901 (accessed July 4, 2016).

ARAÚJO, J. Sousa Soares de; C. Teixeira Regis; R.G. Silva Gomes; T. Ribeiro Tavares; C. Rocha dos Santos; P. Melo Assunção; and R.V. Nóbrega et al. Microcephaly in northeast Brazil: a review of 16 208 births between 2012 and 2015. *Bulletin of the World Health Organization*. February 4, 2016, www.who.int/bulletin/online_first/16-170639.pdf (accessed June 28, 2016).

ATKINSON, Barry; P. Hearn; B. Afrough; S. Lumley; D. Carter; E.J. Aarons; and A.J. Simpson et al. Detection of Zika virus in semen. *Emerging Infectious Diseases*, v. 22, no. 5, p. 940, 2016, www.ncbi.nlm. nih.gov/pmc/articles/PMC4861539/pdf/16-0107.pdf (accessed July 4, 2016).

BALM, Michelle N.D.; C. Kiat Lee; H. Kai Lee; L. Chiu; E.S.C. Koay; and J.W. Tang. A diagnostic polymerase chain reaction assay for Zika virus. *Journal of Medical Virology*, v. 84, no. 9, pp. 1501–1505, 2012, http://onlinelibrary.wiley.com/doi/10.1002/jmv.23241/abstract;jsessio nid=E594BAFC4BCBB2666515671B461708AA.f01t03 (accessed June 28, 2016).

BECKER, Rachel. Missing link: animal models to study whether Zika causes birth defects. *Nature Medicine*, v. 22, no. 3, pp. 225–227, 2016, www. nature.com/doifinder/10.1038/nm0316-225 (accessed June 28, 2016).

BESNARD, M.; S. Lastère; A. Teissier; V.M. Cao-Lormeau; and D. Musso. Evidence of perinatal transmission of Zika virus, French Polynesia, December 2013 and February 2014. *Eurosurveillance*, v. 19, no. 13, pp. 8–11, 2014, www.eurosurveillance.org/images/dynamic/EE/V19N13/ art20751.pdf (accessed July 4, 2016).

BRAGA, Ima Aparecida and D. Valle. Aedes aegypti: histórico do controle no Brasil. *Epidemiologia e Serviços de Saúde*, v. 16, no. 2, pp. 113–118, 2007, http://scielo.iec.pa.gov.br/pdf/ess/v16n2/v16n2a06.pdf (accessed June 28, 2016).

BRITO, Carlos. Zika virus: a new chapter in the history of medicine. *Acta Médica Portuguesa*, v. 28, no. 6, pp. 679–680, 2015, www. actamedicaportuguesa.com/revista/index.php/amp/article/view/7341 (accessed July 4, 2016).

CALVET, G.; R.S. Aguiar; A.S.O. Melo; S.A. Sampaio; I. de Filippis; A. Fabri; and E.S.M. Araujo et al. Detection and sequencing of Zika virus from amniotic fluid of fetuses with microcephaly in Brazil: a case study. *Lancet Infectious Diseases*, pp. 1–8, 2016, www.thelancet.com/ pdfs/journals/laninf/PIIS1473-3099(16)00095-5.pdf (accessed June 28, 2016).

CAMPOS, Gúbio S.; A.C. Bandeira; and S.I. Sardi. Zika virus outbreak, Bahia, Brazil. *Emerging Infectious Diseases*, v. 21, no. 10, pp. 1885–1886, 2015, http://wwwnc.cdc.gov/eid/article/21/10/pdfs/15-0847.pdf (accessed June 28, 2016).

CAMPOS, Gúbio S.; S.I. Sardi; M. Sarno; and C. Brites. Zika virus infection, a new public health challenge. *Brazilian Journal of Infectious Diseases*, v. 20, no. 3, pp. 227–228, 2016, http://dx.doi.org/10.1016/j.bjid.2016.05.001 (accessed June 28, 2016).

CAO-LORMEAU, V.M.; A. Blake; S. Mons; S. Lastère; C. Roche; J. Vanhomwegen; and T. Dub et al. Guillain-Barré Syndrome outbreak caused by Zika virus infection in French Polynesia: a case-control study. *The Lancet*, v. 387, pp. 1531–1539, 2016, www.thelancet.com/ pdfs/journals/lancet/PIIS0140-6736(16)00562-6.pdf (accessed June 28, 2016).

CASSEB, Alexandre do Rosário; L.M. Neves Casseb; S.P da Silva; and P.F. da Costa Vasconcelos. Arbovírus: importante zoonose na Amazônia brasileira. *Veterinária e Zootecnia*, v. 20, no. 3, pp. 9–21, 2013, www. fmvz.unesp.br/rvz/index.php/rvz/article/view/191/461 (accessed June 29, 2016).

CAUCHEMEZ, Simon; M. Besnard; P. Bompard; T. Dub; P. Guillemette-Artur; D. Eyrolle-Guignot; and H. Salje et al. Association between Zika virus and microcephaly in French Polynesia, 2013–15: a retrospective study. *The Lancet*, pp. 1–8, 2016, http://dx.doi.org/10.1016/S0140-6736(16)00651-6 (accessed June 28, 2016).

CAVALCANTI, Luciano Pamplona de Góes; P.L. Tauil; C.H. Alencar; W. Oliveira; M.M. Teixeira; and J. Heukelbach. Zika virus infection, associated microcephaly, and low yellow fever vaccination coverage in

Brazil: is there any causal link? *The Journal of Infection in Developing Countries*, v. 10, no. 6, pp. 563–566, 2016, www.jidc.org/index.php/journal/article/view/8575 (accessed July 18, 2016).

CHAN, Jasper F.W.; G.K.Y. Choi; C.C.Y. Yip; V.C.C. Cheng; and K.-Y. Yuen. Zika fever and congenital Zika syndrome: an unexpected emerging arboviral disease. *Journal of Infection*, v. 72, no. 5, 2016, pp. 507–524, www.journalofinfection.com/article/S0163-4453(16)00061-X/pdf (accessed July 19, 2016).

COELHO, Danilo. Suspeita de Zika no estado. Especialista acredita que a causa das lotações nas emergências seja o vírus. *Folha de Pernambuco*, Recife, May 6, 2015, http://nossavitoriape.com/2015/05/suspeita-de-zika-no-estado.html (accessed June 30, 2016).

COSTA, Federico; M. Sarno; R. Khouri; B. de Paulo Freitas; I. Siqueira; G.S. Ribeiro; and H.C. Ribeiro et al. Emergence of congenital Zika syndrome: viewpoint from the front lines. *Annals of Internal Medicine*, pp. 1–4, 2016, http://annals.org/article.aspx?articleid=2498549 (accessed July 19, 2016).

D'ORTENZIO, Eric; S. Matheron; X. de Lamballerie; B. Hubert; G. Piorkowski; M. Maquart; and D. Descamps et al. Evidence of sexual transmission of Zika virus. *The New England Journal of Medicine*, pp. 1–3, 2016, www.nejm.org/doi/pdf/10.1056/NEJMc1604449 (accessed July 4, 2016).

DAILARD, Cynthia. Understanding "abstinence": implications for individuals, programs and policies. *The Guttmacher Report on Public Policy*, v. 6, no. 5, pp. 4–6, 2003, www.guttmacher.org/sites/default/files/article_files/gr060504.pdf (accessed July 7, 2016).

DECKARD, D. Trew; W.M. Chung; J.T. Brooks; J.C. Smith; S. Woldai; M. Hennessey; N. Kwit; and P. Mead. Male-to-male sexual transmission of Zika virus – Texas, January 2016. *MMWR. Morbidity and Mortality Weekly Report*, v. 65, no. 14, pp. 372–374, 2016, www.ncbi.nlm.nih.gov/pubmed/27078057 (accessed July 4, 2016).

DICK, G.W.A. Zika virus (II). Pathogenicity and physical properties. *Transactions of the Royal Society of Tropical Medicine and Hygiene*, v. 46, no. 5, pp. 521–534, 1952, www.sciencedirect.com/science/article/pii/0035920352900436 (accessed June 29, 2016).

DICK, G.W.A.; S.F. Kitchen; and A.J. Haddow. Zika virus (I). Isolations and serological specificity. *Transactions of the Royal Society of Tropical*

*Medicine and Hygiene*, v. 46, no. 5, pp. 509–520, 1952, trstmh. oxfordjournals.org/content/46/5/509 (accessed June 29, 2016).

DINIZ, Debora. Zika virus and women. *Cadernos de Saúde Pública*, v. 32, no. 5, pp. 1–4, 2016, www.ncbi.nlm.nih.gov/pubmed/27192024 (accessed June 29, 2016).

DINIZ, Debora and Luciana Brito. Epidemia provocada pelo vírus Zika: informação e conhecimento. *Reciis. Revista Eletronica de Comunicação, Informação, Inovação e Saúde*, v. 10, no. 2, pp. 1–5, 2016, www.reciis. icict.fiocruz.br/index.php/reciis/article/view/1148/pdf1148 (accessed July 4, 2016).

DINIZ, Debora and Marcelo Medeiros. Aborto no Brasil: uma pesquisa domiciliar com técnica de urna. *Ciência & Saúde Coletiva*, v. 15, no. 1, pp. 959–966, 2010, www.scielo.br/scielo.php?script=sci_arttext&pid=S1413-81232010000700002 (accessed July 4, 2016).

DUFFY, Mark R.; Tai-Ho Chen; W. Thane Hancock; A.M. Powers; J.L. Kool; R.S. Lanciotti; and M. Pretrick et al. Zika virus outbreak on Yap Island, Federated States of Micronesia. *The New England Journal of Medicine*, v. 360, no. 24, pp. 2536–2543, 2009, www.nejm.org/doi/pdf/10.1056/NEJMoa0805715 (accessed June 29, 2016).

DUPONT-ROUZEYROL, Myrielle; A. Biron; O. O'Connor; E. Huguon; and E. Descloux. Infectious Zika viral particles in breast milk. *The Lancet*, p. 1, 2016, http://linkinghub.elsevier.com/retrieve/pii/S0140673616006243 (accessed June 29, 2016).

DURAND, Mark A.; M. Bel; I. Ruwey; and V. Ngaden. An outbreak of dengue fever in Yap State. *Pacific Health Dialog*, v. 12, no. 2, pp. 99–102, 2005, www.researchgate.net/publication/5667923_An_outbreak_of_dengue_fever_in_Yap_State (accessed July 4, 2016).

FARIA, Nuno Rodrigues; R. do S. da Silva Azevedo; M.U.G. Kraemer; R. Souza; M. Sequetin Cunha; S.C. Hill; and J. Thézé et al. Zika virus in the Americas: early epidemiological and genetic findings. *Science*, v. 352, no. 6283, pp. 345–349, 2016, www.sciencemag.org/cgi/doi/10.1126/science.aaf5036 (accessed June 29, 2016).

FAYE, Oumar; C.C.M. Freire; A. Iamarino; O. Faye; J. Velasco; C. de Oliveira; and M. Diallo et al. Molecular evolution of Zika virus during its emergence in the 20th century. *PLoS Neglected Tropical Diseases*, v. 8, no. 1, p. 36, 2014, www.ncbi.nlm.nih.gov/pmc/articles/PMC3888466/pdf/pntd.0002636.pdf (accessed June 29, 2016).

FOY, Brian D.; K.C. Kobylinski; J.L. Chilson Foy; B.J. Blitvich; A. Travassos da Rosa; A.D. Haddow; R.S. Lanciotti; and R.B. Tesh. Probable non-vector-borne transmission of Zika virus, Colorado, USA. *Emerging Infectious Diseases*, v. 17, no. 5, pp. 880–882, 2011, www.ncbi.nlm.nih.gov/pmc/articles/PMC3321795/pdf/10-1939_finalD.pdf (accessed June 29, 2016).

FRANÇA, Giovanny V.A.; L. Schuler-Faccini; W.K. Oliveira; C.M.P. Henriques; E.H. Carmo; V.D. Pedi; and M.L. Nunes et al. Congenital Zika virus syndrome in Brazil: a case series of the first 1501 live births with complete investigation. *The Lancet*, pp. 1–7, 2016, www.thelancet. com/pdfs/journals/lancet/PIIS0140-6736(16)30902-3.pdf.

FRANK, Christina; M. Faber; and K. Stark. Causal or not: applying the Bradford Hill aspects of evidence to the association between Zika virus and microcephaly. *EMBO Molecular Medicine*, pp. 1–3, 2016, http://onlinelibrary.wiley.com/doi/10.15252/emmm.201506058/pdf (accessed June 29, 2016).

GONZÁLEZ VÉLEZ, Ana Cristina. Comentario sobre el artículo de Baum et al. *Cadernos de Saúde Pública*, Rio de Janeiro, v. 32, no. 5, pp. 1–2, 2016, www.scielo.br/scielo.php?script=sci_arttext&pid=S0102-311X2 016000500606&lng=en&nrm=iso (accessed July 6, 2016).

GRARD, Gilda; M. Caron; I.M. Mombo; D. Nkoghe; S. Mboui Ondo; D. Jiolle; and D. Fontenille et al. Zika virus in Gabon (Central Africa) – 2007: a new threat from Aedes albopictus? *PLoS Neglected Tropical Diseases*, v. 8, no. 2, pp. 1–6, 2014, www.ncbi.nlm.nih.gov/pmc/articles/ PMC3916288/pdf/pntd.0002681.pdf (accessed June 29, 2016).

GRENS, Kerry. Brazil's pre-Zika microcephaly cases. *The Scientist*, February 10, 2016, www.the-scientist.com/?articles.view/articleNo/45297/title/ Brazil-s-Pre-Zika-Microcephaly-Cases/ (accessed June 29, 2016).

GUBLER, Duane J. The global emergence/resurgence of arboviral diseases as public health problems. *Archives of Medical Research*, v. 33, no. 4, pp. 330–342, 2002, www.arcmedres.com/article/S0188-4409(02)00378-8/abstract (accessed June 29, 2016).

GUILLAIN, G.; J.A. Barré; and A. Strohl. Sur un syndrome de radiculonévrite aves hyperalbuminose du liquide céphalo-rachidien sans réaction cellulaire. Remarques sur les caractéres cliniques et graphiques des réflexes tendineux. *Bulletins et mémoires de la Société des Médecins des Hôpitaux de Paris*, Paris, v. 40, pp. 462–470, 1916.

HAYDEN, Erika Check. Spectre of Ebola haunts Zika response. *Nature*, v. 531, p. 19, 2016, www.ncbi.nlm.nih.gov/pubmed/26935676 (accessed July 4, 2016).

HAYES, Edward B. Zika virus outside Africa. *Emerging Infectious Diseases*, v. 15, no. 9, pp. 1347–1350, 2009, http://wwwnc.cdc.gov/eid/article/15/9/pdfs/09-0442.pdf (accessed June 29, 2016).

HONÓRIO, Nildimar Alves; D. Cardoso Portela Câmara; G. Amaral Calvet; and P. Brasil. Chikungunya: an arbovirus infection in the process of establishment and expansion in Brazil. *Cadernos de Saúde Pública*, v. 31, no. 5, pp. 906–908, 2015, www.scielo.br/scielo.php?script=sci_arttext&pid=S0102-311X2015000500003&lng=en&nrm=iso&tlng=en (accessed June 29, 2016).

IOOS, S.; H.-P. Mallet; I.L. Goffart; V. Gauthiera; T. Cardosoa; and M. Herida. Current Zika virus epidemiology and recent epidemics. *Medecine et Maladies Infectieuses*, v. 44, no. 7, pp. 302–307, 2014, http://dx.doi.org/10.1016/j.medmal.2014.04.008 (accessed June 29, 2016).

JOUANNIC, Jean-Marie; S. Friszer; I. Leparc-Goffart; C. Garel; and D. Eyrolle-Guignot. Zika virus infection in French Polynesia. *The Lancet*, pp. 1–2, 2016, www.thelancet.com/journals/lancet/article/PIIS0140-6736(16)00625-5/fulltext?rss=yes (accessed June 29, 2016).

KRAEMER, Moritz U.G.; M.E. Sinka; K.A. Duda; A. Mylne; F.M. Shearer; O.J. Brady; and J.P. Messina et al. The global compendium of Aedes aegypti and Aedes albopictus occurrence. *Science Data*, v. 2, no. 150035, 2015, www.nature.com/articles/sdata201535 (accessed July 7, 2016).

LANCIOTTI, Robert S.; O.L. Kosoy; J.J. Laven; J.O. Velez; A.J. Lambert; A.J. Johnson; S.M. Stanfield; and M.R. Duffy. Genetic and serologic properties of Zika virus associated with an epidemic, Yap State, Micronesia, 2007. *Emerging Infectious Diseases*, v. 14, no. 8, pp. 1232–1239, 2008, www.ncbi.nlm.nih.gov/pubmed/18680646 (accessed June 29, 2016).

LATIN AMERICAN COLLABORATIVE STUDY OF CONGENITAL MALFORMATIONS. *ECLAMC Final Document*. 2015, www.nature.com/polopoly_fs/7.33594!/file/NS-724-2015_ECLAMC-ZIKA VIRUS_V-FINAL_012516.pdf?mbid=synd_msnnews (accessed June 29, 2016).

LOPES, Nayara; C. Nozawa; and R.E.C. Linhares. Características gerais e epidemiologia dos arbovírus emergentes no Brasil. *Revista Pan-Amazônica de Saúde*, v. 5, no. 3, pp. 55–64, 2014, http://scielo.iec.pa.gov.

br/scielo.php?pid=S2176-62232014000300007&script=sci_abstract (accessed June 29, 2016).

LÖWY, Ilana. Zika and microcephaly: can we learn from history? *Physis: Revista de Saúde Coletiva*, v. 26, no. 1, pp. 1–11, 2016a, www.scielo.br/scielo.php?script=sci_arttext&pid=S0103-73312016000100011 (accessed July 4, 2016).

LÖWY, Ilana. Zika virus and rubella: similarities and differences. *História Ciências Saúde - Manguinhos*, 2016b, www.revistahcsm.coc.fiocruz.br/english/zika-virus-an-rubella-similarities-and-differences (accessed July 4, 2016).

MANSUY, Jean Michel; M. Dutertre; C. Mengelle; C. Fourcade; B. Marchou; P. Delobel; J. Izopet; and G. Martin-Blondel. Zika virus: high infectious viral load in semen, a new sexually transmitted pathogen? *The Lancet Infectious Diseases*, v. 16, p. 405, 2016, http://dx.doi.org/10.1016/S1473-3099(16)00138-9 (accessed July 4, 2016).

MARANO, Giuseppe; S. Pupella; S. Vaglio; G.M. Liumbruno; and G. Grazzini. Zika virus and the never-ending story of emerging pathogens and transfusion medicine. *Blood Transfusion*, v. 14, pp. 95–100, 2016, www.bloodtransfusion.it/articolo.aspx?idart=002932&idriv=000108 (accessed June 29, 2016).

MASSAD, Eduardo; F.A. Bezerra Coutinho; and A. Wilder-Smith. Is Zika a substantial risk for visitors to the Rio de Janeiro Olympic Games? *The Lancet*, v. 388, no. 10039, p. 25, 2016, www.thelancet.com/journals/lancet/article/PIIS0140-6736(16)30842-X/fulltext?rss=yes (accessed July 7, 2016).

MELO, Adriana Suely de Oliveira; G. Malinger; R. Ximenes; P.O. Szejnfeld; S. Alves Sampaio; and A.M. Bispo de Filippis. Zika virus intrauterine infection causes fetal brain abnormality and microcephaly: tip of the iceberg? *Ultrasound in Obstetrics and Gynecology*, v. 47, pp. 6–7, 2016, http://onlinelibrary.wiley.com/doi/10.1002/uog.15831/epdf (accessed February 21, 2017).

MIRANDA-FILHO, Demócrito de Barros; C.M. Turchi Martelli; R. Arraes de Alencar Ximenes; T. Velho Barreto Araújo; M.A.W. Rocha; R. Coeli Ferreira Ramos; and R. Dhalia et al. Initial description of the presumed congenital Zika syndrome. *American Journal of Public Health*, v. 106, no. 4, pp. 598–600, 2016, http://ajph.aphapublications.org/doi/pdf/10.2105/AJPH.2016.303115 (accessed June 29, 2016).

MLAKAR, Jernej; M. Korva; N. Tul; M. Popović; M. Poljšak-Prijatelj; J. Mraz; and M. Kolenc et al. Zika virus associated with microcephaly. *The New England Journal of Medicine*, pp. 1–8, 2016, www.nejm.org/doi/abs/10.1056/NEJMoa1600651 (accessed June 29, 2016).

MUSSO, Didier; T. Nhan; E. Robin; C. Roche; D. Bierlaire; K. Zisou; and A. Shan Yan et al. Potential for Zika virus transmission through blood transfusion demonstrated during an outbreak in French Polynesia, November 2013 to February 2014. *Eurosurveillance*, v. 19, no. 14, pp. 1–3, 2014, www.eurosurveillance.org/images/dynamic/EE/V19N14/art20761.pdf (accessed July 4, 2016).

MUSSO, Didier; C. Roche; T. Nhan; E. Robin; A. Teissier; and V.M. Cao-Lormeau. Detection of Zika virus in saliva. *Journal of Clinical Virology: the official publication of the Pan American Society for Clinical Virology*, v. 68, pp. 53–55, 2015a, www.sciencedirect.com/science/article/pii/S1386653215001333X (accessed July 4, 2016).

MUSSO, Didier; C. Roche; E. Robin; T. Nhan; A. Teissier; and V.M. Cao-Lormeau. Potential sexual transmission of Zika virus. *Emerging Infectious Diseases*, v. 21, no. 2, pp. 359–361, 2015b, www.ncbi.nlm.nih.gov/pmc/articles/PMC4313657/ (accessed July 4, 2016).

OEHLER, E.; L. Watrin; P. Larre; I. Leparc-Goffart; S. Lastere; F. Valour; and L. Baudouin et al. Zika virus infection complicated by Guillain-Barré syndrome – case report, French Polynesia, December 2013. *Euro Surveillance: bulletin Européen sur les maladies transmissibles = Euro bulletin*, v. 19, no. 9, pp. 1–2, 2014, www.ncbi.nlm.nih.gov/pubmed/24626205 (accessed June 29, 2016).

PACHECO, Oscar; M. Beltrán; C.A. Nelson; D. Valencia; N. Tolosa; S.L. Farr; and A.V. Padilla et al. Zika virus disease in Colombia: preliminary report. *The New England Journal of Medicine*, pp. 1–10, 2016, www.nejm.org/doi/10.1056/NEJMoa1604037 (accessed July 7, 2016).

PETERSEN, Lyle R.; D.J. Jamieson; A.M. Powers; and M.A. Honein. Zika virus. *The New England Journal of Medicine*, v. 374, pp. 1552–1563, 2016, www.nejm.org/doi/10.1056/NEJMra1602113 (accessed June 28, 2016).

PLOTKIN, Stanley. The history of rubella and rubella vaccination leading to elimination. *Clinical Infectious Diseases*, v. 43, no. 3, November 1, 2006, https://academic.oup.com/cid/article/43/Supplement_3/S164/288915/The-History-of-Rubella-and-Rubella-Vaccination (accessed February 6, 2017).

POLYNÉSIE FRANÇAISE. Direction de la Santé. Centre d'hygiène et de Salubrité Publique de la Direction de la Santé. Surveillance et veille sanitaire en Polynésie française: données du 23 au 29 novembre 2015 (Semaine 48). *Bulletin de Surveillance Sanitaire*, pp. 1–4, 2015, www. hygiene-publique.gov.pf/IMG/pdf/bulletin_surv_pf_sem_48-_2015. pdf (accessed July 12, 2016).

PREIDT, Robert. Zika threat calls for extra mosquito protection this summer. *Medline Plus*, June 2, 2016, www.nlm.nih.gov/medlineplus/ news/fullstory_159168.html (accessed July 5, 2016).

RASMUSSEN, Sonja A.; D.J. Jamieson; M.A. Honein; and L.R. Petersen. Zika virus and birth defects: reviewing the evidence for causality. *The New England Journal of Medicine*, pp. 1–7, 2016, www.nejm.org/doi/ full/10.1056/NEJMsr1604338?query=featured_zika (accessed July 4, 2016).

RODRIGUES, Laura C. Microcephaly and Zika virus infection. *The Lancet*, pp. 1–2, 2016a, http://dx.doi.org/10.1016/S0140-6736(16)00742-X (accessed July 4, 2016).

SAVAGE, H.M.; C.L. Fritz; D. Rutstein; A. Yolwa; V. Vorndam; and D.J. Gubler. Epidemic of Dengue-4 virus in Yap State, Federated States of Micronesia, and implication of Aedes hensilli as an epidemic vector. *The American Journal of Tropical Medicine and Hygiene*, v. 58, no. 4, pp. 519–524, 1998, www.ajtmh.org/content/58/4/519.long (accessed June 29, 2016).

SCHULER-FACCINI, Lavinia; E.M. Ribeiro; I.M.L. Feitosa; D.D.G. Horovitz; D.P. Cavalcanti; A. Pessoa; and M.J.R. Doriqui et al. Possible association between Zika virus infection and microcephaly: Brazil, 2015. *MMWR. Morbidity and Mortality Weekly Report*, v. 65, no. 3, pp. 59–62, 2016, www.cdc.gov/mmwr/volumes/65/wr/mm6503e2. htm (accessed July 4, 2016).

TEIXEIRA, Maria G.; A.M.S. Andrade; M.C.N. Costa; J.S.M. Castro; F.L.S. Oliveira; C.S.B. Goes; and M. Maia et al. East/Central/South African genotype Chikungunya Virus, Brazil, 2014. *Emerging Infectious Diseases*, v. 21, no. 5, pp. 906–908, 2015, http://wwwnc.cdc.gov/eid/ article/21/5/14-1727_article (accessed June 29, 2016).

TURMEL, Jean Marie; P. Abgueguen; Y.M. Vandamme; B. Hubert; M. Maquart; H. Le Guillou-Guillemette; and I. Leparc-Goffart. Late sexual transmission of Zika virus related to persistence in the semen. *The Lancet*, v. 387, p. 2501, 2016, www.thelancet.com/pdfs/journals/ lancet/PIIS0140-6736%2816%2930775-9.pdf (accessed July 4, 2016).

VICTORA, Cesar Gomes; L. Schuler-Faccini; A. Matijasevich; E. Ribeiro; A. Pessoa; and F. Celso Barros. Microcephaly in Brazil: how to interpret reported numbers? *The Lancet*, v. 387, no. 10019, pp. 621–624, 2016, www.sciencedirect.com/science/article/pii/S0140673616002737 (accessed June 29, 2016).

VOGEL, Gretchen. Don't blame sports for Zika's spread. *Science*, v. 351, no. 6280, pp. 1377–1378, 2016a, http://science.sciencemag.org/content/351/6280/1377?utm_campaign=email-sci-toc&et_rid=34807268&et_cid=364259 (accessed June 29, 2016).

VOGEL, Gretchen. Zika virus discovered in infant brains bolsters link to microcephaly. *Science*, February 11, 2016b, www.sciencemag.org/news/2016/02/zika-virus-discovered-infant-brains-bolsters-link-microcephaly (accessed June 29, 2016).

YUKI, Nobuhiro and H.-P. Hartung. Guillain-Barré Syndrome. *The New England Journal of Medicine*, v. 366, no. 24, pp. 2294–2304, 2012, www.nejm.org/doi/abs/10.1056/NEJMra1114525 (accessed June 30, 2016).

ZANLUCA, Camila and C.N. Duarte dos Santos. Zika virus: an overview. *Microbes and Infection*, pp. 1–7, 2016, http://linkinghub.elsevier.com/retrieve/pii/S1286457916000496 (accessed June 30, 2016).

ZANLUCA, Camila; V. Campos Andrade de Melo; A.L. Pamplona Mosimann; G.I. Viana dos Santos; C.N. Duarte dos Santos; and K. Luz. First report of autochthonous transmission of Zika virus in Brazil. *Memórias do Instituto Oswaldo Cruz*, v. 110, no. 4, pp. 569–572, 2015, www.ncbi.nlm.nih.gov/pubmed/26061233 (accessed June 30, 2016).

ZHU, Zheng; J. Fuk-Woo Chan; Kah-Meng Tee; G. Kwan-Yue Choi; S. Kar-Pui Lau; P. Chiu-Yat Woo; H. Tse; and Kwok-Yung Yuen. Comparative genomic analysis of pre-epidemic and epidemic Zika virus strains for virological factors potentially associated with the rapidly expanding epidemic. *Emerging Microbes & Infections*, v. 5, no. e22, pp. 1–11, July 7, 2016, www.nature.com/emi/journal/v5/n3/pdf/emi201648a.pdf (accessed July 7, 2016).

## NEWSPAPER AND MAGAZINE ARTICLES, BLOG POSTS

AGÊNCIA da ONU propõe esterilizar Aedes aegypti com radiação. *G1*, February 2, 2016, http://g1.globo.com/bemestar/noticia/2016/02/

agencia-da-onu-propoe-esterilizar-aedes-aegypti-com-radiacao.html
(accessed July 13, 2016).

AZEVEDO, Ana Lucia. "Estamos com os pés e mãos atados," diz médico
sobre Zika. *O Globo*, Rio de Janeiro, December 5, 2015, http://oglobo.
globo.com/sociedade/saude/estamos-com-os-pes-maos-atados-diz-
medico-sobre-zika-18227041 (accessed July 4, 2016).

BACTÉRIA diminui capacidade de Aedes transmitir o vírus da Zika. *G1 São
Paulo*, May 4, 2016, http://g1.globo.com/bemestar/noticia/2016/05/
bacteria-diminui-capacidade-de-aedes-transmitir-o-virus-da-zika.
html (accessed July 13, 2016).

BAJAJ, Vikas. How Zika became a global threat. *The New York Times*, June
13, 2016, http://takingnote.blogs.nytimes.com/2016/06/13/how-zika-
became-a-global-threat/ (accessed July 5, 2016).

BARATA, Germana. Primeira descrição do zika vírus transmitido no país
alerta para crescimento da doença. *Divulga Ciência*, June 19, 2015,
https://blogdivulgaciencia.wordpress.com/2015/06/19/primeira-
descricao-de-casos-do-zika-virus-transmitidos-no-pais-alerta-para-
crescimento-da-doenca/ (accessed July 13, 2016).

BORGES, Taiana. Pesquisadores criam biolarvicida que elimina as larvas
do Aedes Aegypti. *EBC Rádios*, Brasilia, June 16, 2016, http://radios.
ebc.com.br/amazonia-brasileira/edicao/2016-06/pesquisadores-criam-
biolarvicida-capaz-de-eliminar-larvas-do (accessed July 13, 2016).

BRASIL não registrava microcefalia, diz vice-ministro de saúde da
Colômbia. *Zero Hora*, March 3, 2016, http://zh.clicrbs.com.br/rs/vida-
e-estilo/vida/noticia/2016/03/brasil-nao-registrava-microcefalia-diz-
vice-ministro-de-saude-da-colombia-4991937.html (accessed June 30,
2016).

BUCCI, Steven. It's time for the world to take the Zika threat seriously.
*The Daily Signal*, June 9, 2016, http://dailysignal.com/2016/06/09/its-
time-for-the-world-to-take-the-zika-threat-seriously/ (accessed July
5, 2016).

CANCIAN. Natália. Anvisa dará aval temporário a pesquisas com aedes
transgênico. *Folha de S. Paulo*, April 12, 2016, http://www1.folha.uol.
com.br/cotidiano/2016/04/1759901-anvisa-dara-aval-temporario-a-
pesquisas-com-aedes-transgenico.shtml (accessed July 13, 2016).

CASOS de microcefalia foram subnotificados na "era pré Zika," mostram
estudos. *Veja*, São Paulo, February 15, 2016, http://veja.abril.com.br/

saude/casos-de-microcefalia-foram-subnotificados-na-era-pre-zika-mostram-estudos (accessed June 29, 2016).

CIENTISTAS do Instituto Pasteur estão no Brasil para combater o Zika vírus. *USP – Sala de Imprensa*, São Paulo, January 7, 2016, www.usp.br/imprensa/?p=54787 (accessed June 30, 2016).

COGHLAN, Andy. Whole Zika genome recovered from brain of baby with microcephaly. *New Scientist*, February 10, 2016, www.newscientist.com/article/2077091-whole-zika-genome-recovered-from-brain-of-baby-with-microcephaly (accessed June 28, 2016).

COSTA, Camilla. Gêmeo com irmão saudável foi "paciente zero" em epidemia de microcefalia, diz médica. *BBC Brasil*, December 4, 2015, www.bbc.com/portuguese/noticias/2015/12/151204_microcefalia_paciente_zero_cc (accessed June 28, 2016).

COSTA, Catarina. Pesquisa descobre planta típica do PI capaz de combater o Aedes aegypti. *G1 Piauí*, February 15, 2016, http://g1.globo.com/pi/piaui/noticia/2016/02/pesquisa-descobre-planta-tipica-do-pi-capaz-de-combater-o-aedes-aegypti.html (accessed July 13, 2016).

COSTA JUNIOR, Jairo. Diagnósticos de casos de Zika na Bahia podem estar errados. *Correio da Bahia*, May 8, 2015, www.correio24horas.com.br/detalhe/noticia/satelite-diagnosticos-de-casos-de-zika-na-bahia-podem-estar-errados/?cHash=cd6b57743d456ded02775c03f5e773ad (accessed June 29, 2016).

CREMEPE cria câmara sobre microcefalia. *Jornal do Commercio*, Recife, October 27, 2015, http://jconline.ne10.uol.com.br/canal/cidades/saude/noticia/2015/10/27/cremepe-cria-camara-tematica-de-microcefalia-205345.php (accessed June 29, 2016).

DALTON, Juan José. Zika vírus faz El Salvador recomendar que mulheres evitem gravidez até 2018. *El País*, January 27, 2016, http://brasil.elpais.com/brasil/2016/01/26/internacional/1453844344_353247.html (accessed July 8, 2016).

DOENÇA misteriosa em Camaçari pode ser roséola ou parvovírus. *A Tarde*, Salvador, March 25, 2015, http://atarde.uol.com.br/bahia/noticias/1669487-doenca-misteriosa-em-camacari-pode-ser-roseola-ou-parvovirus (accessed June 28, 2016).

DOIS casos de febre Chikungunya são confirmados no Rio de Janeiro. *G1 Rio*, Rio de Janeiro, July 7, 2014, http://g1.globo.com/rio-de-janeiro/noticia/2014/07/dois-casos-de-febre-chikungunya-sao-confirmados-no-rj.html (accessed June 29, 2016).

EL ZIKA ¿Una amenaza global? *Eitb.eus*, April 15, 2016, www.eitb. eus/es/radio/radio-euskadi/programas/la-mecanica-del-caracol/ detalle/3988648/el-zika-una-amenaza-global/ (accessed July 5, 2016).

ESTUDO propõe edição genética para eliminar fêmeas de Aedes aegypti. *G1*, February 18, 2016, http://g1.globo.com/ciencia-e-saude/noticia/ 2016/02/estudo-propoe-edicao-genetica-para-eliminar-femeas-de-aedes-aegypti.html (accessed July 13, 2016).

EXAMES confirmam infecção por Zika vírus em dois casos de microcefalia. *G1 Paraíba*, November 17, 2015, http://g1.globo.com/pb/paraiba/ noticia/2015/11/exames-comprovam-infeccao-por-zika-virus-em-dois-casos-de-microcefalia.html (accessed June 29, 2016).

FORMENTI, Ligia. Conversa entre médicas provocou alerta sobre microcefalia. *O Estado de S. Paulo*, São Paulo, November 12, 2015a, http://saude.estadao.com.br/noticias/geral,conversa-entre-medicas-provocou-alerta-sobre-microcefalia,10000001774 (accessed June 29, 2016).

FORMENTI, Ligia. "Sexo é para amadores, gravidez é para profissionais," diz ministro da Saúde. *O Estado de S. Paulo*, November 18, 2015b, http:// saude.estadao.com.br/noticias/geral,sexo-e-para-amadores-gravidez-e-para-profissionais-diz-ministro da-saude,10000002325 (accessed June 29, 2016).

FORMENTI, Ligia. Governo confirma zika em dois casos de microcefalia. *O Estado de S Paulo*, São Paulo, November 17, 2015c. http://saude. estadao.com.br/noticias/geral,governo-confirma-zika-em-dois-casos-de-microcefalia,10000002227?success=true (accessed February 16, 2017).

FORMENTI, Lígia. Vice-ministro de Saúde da Colômbia: "Brasil não registrava microcefalia." *O Estado de S. Paulo*, São Paulo, March 7, 2016, http://saude.estadao.com.br/noticias/geral,historicamente-o-brasil-nao-registrava-microcefalia--diz-vice-ministro-de-saude-da-colombia,1840461 (accessed July 5, 2016).

FRANCO, Marcella. Síndrome paralisante faz quarta vítima no Brasil. *R7 Notícias*, São Paulo, July 25, 2015, http://noticias.r7.com/saude/ sindrome-paralisante-faz-quarta-vitima-no-brasil-25072015 (accessed June 29, 2016).

GERMANO, Felipe. 10 heróis que marcaram 2015. *Superinteressante*, São Paulo, December 20, 2015, http://super.abril.com.br/comportamento/ 10-herois-que-marcaram-2015 (accessed June 29, 2016).

GIL, Felipe Salazar. Esperamos 300 casos de microcefalia asociados a zika este año. *El País*, June 23, 2016, www.elpais.com.co/cali/esperamos-300-casos-de-microcefalia-asociados-a-zika-este-ano-ins.html (accessed June 30, 2016).

GOODMAN, Joshua and M. Savarese. Zika: Brasil lucha contra falta de recursos e inoperancia. *Associated Press*, March 18, 2016, http://noticias. terra.cl/mundo/zika-brasil-lucha-contra-falta-de-recursos-e-inoperan cia,87b356f83b2370bb1c7eba4f8dad5975g7akavec.html (accessed July 4, 2016).

GRAIL, Ann. Zika virus: emerging threat catches the world unprepared. *Thomson Reuters*, [2016], http://stateofinnovation.thomsonreuters. com/zika-virus-emerging-threat-catches-the-world-unprepared (accessed July 5, 2016).

IDENTIFICADO vírus causador de doença misteriosa em Salvador E RMS. *G1 Bahia*, Salvador, April 29, 2015, http://g1.globo.com/bahia/ noticia/2015/04/identificado-virus-causador-de-doenca-misteriosa-em-salvador-e-rms.html (accessed June 29, 2016).

JORNAL DA CORREIO. Esclarecimentos sobre microcefalia e Zika vírus: entrevista com Dra. Adriana Melo. February 19, 2016, http://vimow. com/br/watch/x3e45kp_Jornal+da+Correio+-+ESCLARECIMEN TOS+SOBRE+MICROCEFALIA+E+ZIKA+V%C3%8DRUS+-+ENTREVISTA+-+DRA+ADRIANA+MELO (accessed February 23, 2017).

KASSAM, Ashifa. Zika virus makes Rio Olympics a threat in Brazil and abroad, health expert says. *The Guardian*, May 12, 2016, www. theguardian.com/world/2016/may/12/rio-olympics-zika-amir-attaran-public-health-threat (accessed July 5, 2016).

LEITE, Cynthia. Força-tarefa investiga microcefalia em Pernambuco. *Jornal do Commercio*, Recife, October 24, 2015, http://jconline.ne10.uol. com.br/canal/cidades/saude/noticia/2015/10/24/forca-tarefa-investiga-microcefalia-em-pernambuco--205072.php (accessed June 29, 2016).

LENHARO, Mariana. Febre Chikungunya tem sinais que lembram dengue; conheça a doença. *G1 São Paulo*, São Paulo, July 8, 2014, http:// g1.globo.com/bemestar/noticia/2014/07/chikungunya-tem-sintomas-parecidos-com-dengue-conheca-doenca.html (accessed June 29, 2016).

MCNEIL JR., Donald G. Sex may spread Zika virus more often than researchers suspected. *The New York Times*, July 2, 2016, www.

nytimes.com/2016/07/05/health/zika-virus-sex-spread.html?hpw
&rref=health&action=click&pgtype=Homepage&module=well-
region&region=bottom-well&WT.nav=bottom-well&_r=0 (accessed
July 7, 2016).

MELO, Ruan. Doença sem diagnóstico assusta moradores de Camaçari:
angustiante. *G1 Bahia*, Salvador, March 24, 2015, http://g1.globo.com/
bahia/noticia/2015/03/doenca-sem-diagnostico-assusta-moradores-
de-camacari-angustiante.html (accessed June 29, 2016).

MICROCEFALIA: Pernambuco sensibiliza especialistas de outros estados a
ficarem atentos à malformação. *Jornal do Commercio*, Recife, November
13, 2015, http://jconline.ne10.uol.com.br/canal/cidades/saude/noticia/
2015/11/13/microcefalia-pernambuco-sensibiliza-especialistas-de-
outros-estados-a-ficarem-atentos-a-malformacao-207844.php
(accessed June 28, 2016).

MINISTÉRIO da Saúde confirma relação entre microcefalia e o vírus da
Zika. *G1 Brasilia*, November 28, 2015, http://g1.globo.com/bemestar/
noticia/2015/11/ministerio-da-saude-confirma-relacao-entre-
microcefalia-e-virus-zika.html (accessed July 4, 2016).

PE tem situação de emergência e PB também tem casos de microcefalia.
*PB Agora*, João Pessoa, November 11, 2015, www.pbagora.com.br/
conteudo.php?id=20151111215928&cat=saude&keys=pe-tem-situacao-
emergencia-pb-tambem-tem-casos-microcefalia (accessed July 4,
2016).

POPE: Contraceptives could be morally permissible in avoiding spread of
Zika. *The Washington Post*, February 18, 2016, www.washingtonpost.
com/local/social-issues/pope-contraceptives-could-be-morally-
permissable-in-avoiding-spread-of-zika/2016/02/18/64d029de-d673-
11e5-be55-2cc3c1e4b76b_story.html?utm_term=.6a4df967ba38 (accessed
March 3, 2017).

REINACH, Fernando. Microcefalia que sempre existiu. *O Estado de S. Paulo*,
São Paulo, February 6, 2016a, http://saude.estadao.com.br/noticias/
geral,microcefalia-que-sempre-existiu,10000015230 (accessed June 29,
2016).

REINACH, Fernando. Microcefalia: Dados Sumiram. *O Estado de S.
Paulo*, São Paulo, February 20, 2016b, http://saude.estadao.com.br/
noticias/geral,microcefalia-dados-sumiram,10000017316 (accessed June
29, 2016).

REINACH, Fernando. Microcefalia: falta o denominador. *O Estado de S. Paulo*, São Paulo, February 13, 2016c, http://saude.estadao.com.br/noticias/geral,microcefalia-falta-o-denominador,10000016105 (accessed June 29, 2016).

RESK, Felipe. Homens abandonam mães de bebês com microcefalia em PE. *O Estado de S. Paulo*, São Paulo, February 4, 2016, http://saude.estadao.com.br/noticias/geral,homens-abandonam-maes-de-bebes-com-microcefalia-em-pe,10000014877 (accessed July 4, 2016).

RODRIGUES, Ana Helena. 4 motivos para não acreditar no boato que liga vacinas vencidas ao zika vírus. *Época*, December 10, 2015, http://epoca.globo.com/vida/noticia/2015/12/4-motivos-para-nao-acreditar-no-boato-que-liga-vacinas-vencidas-ao-zika-virus.html (accessed July 13, 2016).

RODRIGUES, Léo. Pesquisa comprova eficácia de óleos de orégano e de cravo no combate ao Aedes. *EBC Agência Brasil*, Brasilia, March 14, 2016b, http://agenciabrasil.ebc.com.br/pesquisa-e-inovacao/noticia/2016-03/pesquisa-comprova-eficacia-de-oleos-de-oregano-e-de-cravo-no (accessed July 13, 2016).

SALZBERG, Steven. The Zika virus poses a threat to everyone, especially at the Rio Olympics. *Forbes*, June 20, 2016, www.forbes.com/sites/stevensalzberg/2016/06/20/the-zika-virus-poses-a-threat-to-everyone-especially-at-the-rio-olympics/#2cd0a9364c7c (accessed July 5, 2016).

SANTORA, Marc. As Zika threat grows in U.S., testing lags for a vulnerable group. *The New York Times*, June 17, 2016, www.nytimes.com/2016/06/18/nyregion/zika-testing-lags-in-a-vulnerable-new-york-population.html?_r=0 (accessed July 5, 2016).

SENRA, Ricardo. Grupo prepara ação no STF por aborto em casos de microcefalia. *BBC Brasil*, January 29, 2016, www.bbc.com/portuguese/noticias/2016/01/160126_zika_stf_pai_rs (accessed June 29, 2016).

SINGER, Peter. Given the Zika threat, should the world go to Rio? *The Japan Times*, June 14, 2016, www.japantimes.co.jp/opinion/2016/06/14/commentary/world-commentary/given-zika-threat-world-go-rio/#.V3yKc5MrJmB (accessed July 5, 2016).

TOLEDO, Karina. Risco de contrair Zika durante as Olimpíadas divide especialistas. *Pesquisa Fapesp*, June 1, 2016, http://revistapesquisa.fapesp.br/2016/06/01/risco-de-contrair-zika-durante-as-olimpiadas-divide-especialistas/ (accessed July 5, 2016).

TV NBR. Brasileiros ocupam 100% das vagas ofertadas pelo programa Mais Médicos, May 14, 2015, www.youtube.com/watch?v=8w4YlEKjm_U (accessed June 30, 2016).

URUGUAI registra 1º caso de vírus zika; vírus teria sido contraído no Brasil. *G1 São Paulo*, April 6, 2016, http://g1.globo.com/bemestar/noticia/2016/04/uruguai-registra-1-caso-de-zika-virus-teria-sido-contraido-no-brasil.html (accessed July 7, 2016).

VILLELA, Sumaia. Pesquisadores usam radiação para impedir reprodução do Aedes aegypti. *EBC Agência Brasil*, Brasilia, February 16, 2016, http://agenciabrasil.ebc.com.br/pesquisa-e-inovacao/noticia/2016-02/pesquisadores-usam-radiacao-para-impedir-reproducao-do-aedes (accessed July 13, 2016).

WILLETS, Melissa. It's almost mosquito season: how is the U.S. prepping for the Zika threat? *Parents*, [2016], www.parents.com/health/parents-news-now/its-almost-mosquito-season-how-is-the-us-prepping-for-the-zika-threat/ (accessed July 5, 2016).

XAVIER, Gustavo. "Ainda choro muito," diz grávida de bebê com microcefalia na Paraíba. *G1 Paraíba*, December 11, 2015, http://g1.globo.com/pb/paraiba/noticia/2015/12/ainda-choro-muito-diz-gravida-de-bebe-com-microcefalia-na paraiba.html (accessed February 22, 2017).

## GOVERNMENT

BAHIA. Secretaria da Saúde do Estado da Bahia. *Nota técnica n. 03/2015 – DIVEP/LACEN/SUVISA/SESA*. Salvador: Secretaria da Saúde, 2015, www.saude.ba.gov.br/novoportal/images/stories/PDF/NOTATECNICA_ZIKA_DEI_18062015_%20revisada%20SUVISA%20pdf.pdf (accessed June 29, 2016).

BRASIL. Ministério da Saúde. Portaria nº 104, de 25 de janeiro de 2011. Define as terminologias adotadas em legislação nacional, conforme o disposto no Regulamento Sanitário Internacional 2005 (RSI 2005), a relação de doenças, agravos e eventos em saúde pública de notificação compulsória em todo o território nacional e estabelece fluxo, critérios, responsabilidades e atribuições aos profissionais e serviços de saúde. *Diário Oficial [da União]*, Brasilia, DF, January 26, 2011, http://bvsms.saude.gov.br/bvs/saudelegis/gm/2011/prt0104_25_01_2011.html (accessed July 4, 2016).

BRASIL. Ministério da Saúde. Portaria nº 1.813 de 11 de novembro de 2015. Declara Emergência em Saúde Pública de importância Nacional (ESPIN) por alteração do padrão de ocorrência de microcefalias no Brasil. *Diário Oficial [da União]*, Brasilia, DF, November 12, 2015a, http://www.poderesaude.com.br/novosite/images/publicacoes_ 12.11.2015-II.pdf (accessed June 29, 2016).

BRASIL. Ministério da Saúde. Ministério da Saúde confirma relação entre vírus Zika e microcefalia. *Portal da Saúde*, Brasilia, November 28, 2015b, http://portalsaude.saude.gov.br/index.php/cidadao/principal/agencia-saude/21014-ministerio-da-saude-confirma-relacao-entre-virus-zika-e-microcefalia (accessed June 28, 2016).

BRASIL. Ministério da Saúde. Ministério da Saúde divulga novos dados de microcefalia. *Portal da Saúde*, Brasilia, December 1, 2015c, http://portalsaude.saude.gov.br/index.php/cidadao/principal/ agencia-saude/21019-ministerio-da-saude-divulga-novos-dados-de-microcefalia (accessed June 28, 2016).

BRASIL. Ministério da Saúde. Portaria nº 204, de 17 de fevereiro de 2016. Define a Lista Nacional de Notificação Compulsória de doenças, agravos e eventos de saúde pública nos serviços de saúde públicos e privados em todo o território nacional, nos termos do anexo, e dá outras providências. *Diário Oficial [da União]*, Brasilia, DF, February 18, 2016a, http://portalpbh.pbh.gov.br/pbh/ecp/files.do?evento=down load&urlArqPlc=portaria204-17-fevereiro-2016.pdf (accessed June 28, 2016).

BRASIL. Ministério da Saúde. *Protocolo para implantação de unidades sentinelas para Zika vírus*. Brasilia: Ministério da Saúde, 2016b, http:// portalsaude.saude.gov.br/images/pdf/2015/dezembro/14/Protocolo-Unidades-Sentinela-Zika-v--rus.pdf (accessed June 28, 2016).

BRASIL. Ministério da Saúde. *Zika zero*. Brasilia: Ministério da Saúde, 2016c, http://189.28.128.100/dab/docs/portaldab/documentos/zica_zero. pdf (accessed July 8, 2016).

BRASIL. Ministério da Saúde. Centro de Operações de Emergências em Saúde Pública sobre Microcefalias. *Informe epidemiológico n. 01/2015, Semana Epidemiológica 46 (15 a 21/11/2015): monitoramento dos casos de microcefalia no Brasil*, 2015a, http://portalsaude.saude.gov.br/images/ pdf/2015/novembro/24/COES-Microcefalias---Informe-Epidemiol--gico---SE-46---24nov2015.pdf (accessed July 4, 2016).

# BIBLIOGRAPHY

BRASIL. Ministério da Saúde. Centro de Operações de Emergências em Saúde Pública sobre Microcefalias. *Informe epidemiológico n. 06/2015, Semana Epidemiológica 51 (20 a 26/12/2015): monitoramento dos casos de microcefalias no Brasil,* 2015b, http://portalarquivos.saude.gov. br/images/pdf/2015/dezembro/30/COES-Microcefalias---Informe-Epidemiol--gico---SE-51---29dez2015---15h.pdf (accessed February 24, 2017).

BRASIL. Ministério da Saúde. Centro de Operações de Emergências em Saúde Pública sobre Microcefalias. *Informe epidemiológico n. 32, Semana Epidemiológica 25/2016 (19/06 a 25/06/2016): monitoramento dos casos de microcefalia no Brasil,* 2016a, http://combateaedes.saude.gov.br/images/ pdf/informe_microcefalia_epidemiologico_32.pdf (accessed July 8, 2016).

BRASIL. Ministério da Saúde. Centro de Operações de Emergências em Saúde Pública sobre Microcefalias. *Informe epidemiológico no. 34, Semana Epidemiológica (SE) 27/2016 (03/07 a 09/07/2016): monitoramento dos casos de microcefalia no Brasil,* 2016b, http://combateaedes.saude.gov. br/images/pdf/informe_microcefalia_epidemiologico34.pdf (accessed July 15, 2016).

BRASIL. Ministério da Saúde. Secretaria de Vigilância em Saúde. Monitoramento dos casos de dengue Semana Epidemiológica (SE) 35 e febre de chikungunya SE 36 de 2014. *Boletim Epidemiológico,* v. 45, no. 20, pp. 1 6, 2014, http://portalsaude.saude.gov.br/images/pdf/2014/ setembro/30/BE-2014-45--20----Dengue--SE35--e-CHIKV--SE36-.pdf (accessed June 29, 2016).

BRASIL. Ministério da Saúde. Secretaria de Vigilância em Saúde. *Protocolo de vigilância e resposta à ocorrência de microcefalia relacionada à infecção pelo vírus Zika.* Brasilia: Ministério da Saúde, 2015, http://portalsaude. saude.gov.br/images/pdf/2015/dezembro/09/Microcefalia---Protocolo-de-vigil--ncia-e-resposta---vers--o-1----09dez2015-8h.pdf (accessed June 28, 2016).

BRASIL. Ministério da Saúde. Secretaria de Vigilância em Saúde. *Protocolo de vigilância e resposta à ocorrência de microcefalia e/ou alterações do sistema nervoso central (SNC).* Brasilia: Ministério da Saúde, 2016a, http:// portalsaude.saude.gov.br/images/pdf/2016/marco/10/microcefalia-protocolo-vigilancia-resposta-v2-10mar2016.pdf (accessed June 29, 2016).

BRASIL. Ministério da Saúde. Secretaria de Vigilância em Saúde. Monitoramento dos casos de dengue, febre de chikungunya e febre pelo vírus Zika até a Semana Epidemiológica 20, 2016. *Boletim Epidemiológico*, v. 47, no. 26, pp. 1–10, 2016b, http://combateaedes. saude.gov.br/images/boletins-epidemiologicos/2016-Dengue_Zika_ Chikungunya-SE20.pdf (accessed July 15, 2016).

COLOMBIA. Corte Constitucional de Colombia. Sentencia nº C-355/06. Demandante: Mónica del Pilar Roa López e outros. Demandas de inconstitucionalidad contra los Arts. 122, 123 (parcial), 124, modificados por el Art. 14 de la Ley 890 de 2004, y 32, numeral 7, de la ley 599 de 2000 Código Penal. Relatores: Magistrados Jaime Araújo Rentería e Clara Inés Vargas Hernandez. Corte Constitucional de Colombia. Bogotá, D.C., 2006, www.corteconstitucional.gov.co/relatoria/2006/ c-355-06.htm (accessed July 7, 2016).

INSTITUTO EVANDRO CHAGAS. Apresentação, [n.d.], www.iec.pa.gov.br/ index.php/gcPagina/index/296?semMenu=true (accessed July 5, 2016).

INSTITUTO EVANDRO CHAGAS. IEC comprova relação do vírus Zika com a microcefalia e diagnostica os primeiros óbitos relacionados ao vírus. Instituto Evandro Chagas, December 18, 2015, www.iec.gov.br/index. php/destaque/index/762 (accessed July 4, 2016).

INSTITUTO OSWALDO CRUZ. IOC/FIOCRUZ identifica a presença de Zika vírus em dois casos de microcefalia. *Portal Fiocruz*, November 18, 2015, http://portal.fiocruz.br/pt-br/content/iocfiocruz-identifica-presenca- de-zika-virus-em-dois-casos-de-microcefalia (accessed July 4, 2016).

PERNAMBUCO. Secretaria Estadual de Saúde. Secretaria Executiva de Vigilância em Saúde. *Nota Técnica Nº 59 de 2015. Circulação da febre Zika vírus em Pernambuco. Orientações para vigilância e para a assistência à saúde.* Recife: Secretaria de Saúde, 2015a, http://media.wix.com/ ugd/3293a8_f92bc15b06f64e26806397c579c4401b.pdf (accessed June 30, 2016).

PERNAMBUCO. Secretaria Estadual de Saúde. Secretaria Executiva de Vigilância em Saúde. PE investirá R$ 25 milhões contra Aedes aegypti. *Portal da Saúde*, Recife, November 30, 2015b, http://portal.saude. pe.gov.br/noticias/secretaria/pe-investira-r-25-milhoes-contra-aedes- aegypti (accessed July 12, 2016).

PERNAMBUCO. Secretaria Estadual de Saúde. Secretaria Executiva de Vigilância em Saúde. *Protocolo clínico e epidemiológico para investigação de casos de microcefalia no estado de Pernambuco,* 2015c, http://media. wix.com/ugd/3293a8_bdbc939959174a79941f197903ad3bc9.pdf (accessed June 30, 2016).

PERNAMBUCO. Secretaria Estadual de Saúde. Secretaria Executiva de Vigilância em Saúde. *Nota Técnica SEVS/DGCDA n° 43/15.* Recife: Secretaria de Saúde, 2015d, http://media.wix.com/ugd/3293a8_9dd502 333c274e359226be4cd95598b7.pdf (accessed July 4, 2016).

## CDC/PAHO/WHO

CENTERS FOR DISEASE CONTROL AND PREVENTION. *Arbovirus Catalog,* [n.d.], https://wwwn.cdc.gov/Arbocat/Default.aspx (accessed June 28, 2016).

CENTERS FOR DISEASE CONTROL AND PREVENTION. Guidelines for travelers visiting friends and family in areas with Chikungunya, Dengue, or Zika. June 16, 2016a, http://wwwnc.cdc.gov/travel/page/ guidelines-vfr-chikungunya-dengue-zika (accessed July 7, 2016).

CENTERS FOR DISEASE CONTROL AND PREVENTION. All countries and territories with active Zika virus transmission. June 30, 2016b, www. cdc.gov/zika/geo/active-countries.html (accessed July 7, 2016).

CENTERS FOR DISEASE CONTROL AND PREVENTION. Zika and sexual transmission. July 1, 2016c, www.cdc.gov/zika/transmission/sexual transmission.html (accessed July 7, 2016).

PAN AMERICAN HEALTH ORGANIZATION. *Epidemiological Alert: neurological syndrome, congenital malformations, and Zika virus infection. Implications for public health in the Americas.* Washington, DC: PAHO, 2015, www. paho.org/hq/index.php?option=com_docman&task=doc_view&Itemi d=270&gid=32405&lang=en (accessed June 29, 2016).

PAN AMERICAN HEALTH ORGANIZATION. *Guideline for surveillance of Zika virus disease and its complications.* Washington, DC: PAHO, 2016a, http://iris.paho.org/xmlui/bitstream/handle/123456789/28405/97892751 18948_eng.pdf?sequence=1&isAllowed=y (accessed June 29, 2016).

PAN AMERICAN HEALTH ORGANIZATION. *Lineamentos preliminares de vigilancia de microcefalia en recién nacidos en entornos con riesgo de circulación de virus Zika.* Washington, DC, 2016b, PAHO, www.paho. org/hq/index.php?option=com_docman&task=doc_view&Itemid=270 &gid=32999 (accessed June 29, 2016).

PAN AMERICAN HEALTH ORGANIZATION. *Zika ethics consultation: ethics guidance on key issues raised by the outbreak.* Washington, DC: PAHO, 2016c, http://iris.paho.org/xmlui/bitstream/handle/123456789/28425/PAHOKBR16002_eng.pdf (accessed June 29, 2016).

WHO SCIENTIFIC GROUP. *Arthropod-borne and rodent-borne viral diseases.* Geneva: World Health Organization, 1985, http://apps.who.int/iris/bitstream/10665/39922/1/WHO_TRS_719.pdf (accessed June 30, 2016).

WORLD HEALTH ORGANIZATION. Swine influenza. Geneva: World Health Organization, April 25, 2009, www.who.int/mediacentre/news/statements/2009/h1n1_20090425/en/ (accessed July 7, 2016).

WORLD HEALTH ORGANIZATION. WHO statement on the meeting of the International Health Regulations Emergency Committee concerning the international spread of wild poliovirus. Geneva: World Health Organization, May 5, 2014a, www.who.int/mediacentre/news/statements/2014/polio-20140505/en/ (accessed July 7, 2016).

WORLD HEALTH ORGANIZATION. Statement on the 1st meeting of the IHR Emergency Committee on the 2014 Ebola outbreak in West Africa. Geneva: World Health Organization, August 8, 2014b, www.who.int/mediacentre/news/statements/2014/ebola-20140808/en/ (accessed July 7, 2016).

WORLD HEALTH ORGANIZATION. *Developing global norms for sharing data and results during public health emergencies.* Geneva: World Health Organization, 2015, www.who.int/medicines/ebola-treatment/data-sharing_phe/en/ (accessed June 30, 2016).

WORLD HEALTH ORGANIZATION. *Zika situation report:* Zika virus, microcephaly and Guillain-Barré syndrome. Geneva: World Health Organization, April 7, 2016a, www.who.int/emergencies/zika-virus/situation-report/7-april-2016/en/ (accessed June 29, 2016).

WORLD HEALTH ORGANIZATION. WHO confirms Zika virus strain imported from the Americas to Cabo Verde. Geneva: World Health Organization, May 20, 2016b, www.who.int/mediacentre/news/releases/2016/zika-cabo-verde/en/ (accessed July 7, 2016).

WORLD HEALTH ORGANIZATION. *Prevention of sexual transmission of Zika virus*: interim guidance update. Geneva: World Health Organization, June 7, 2016c, http://apps.who.int/iris/bitstream/10665/204421/1/WHO_ZIKV_MOC_16.1_eng.pdf (accessed July 5, 2016).

WORLD HEALTH ORGANIZATION. WHO statement on the third meeting of the International Health Regulations (2005) (IHR 2005) Emergency committee on Zika vírus and observed increase in neurological disorders and neonatal malformations. Geneva: World Health Organization, June 14, 2016d, www.who.int/mediacentre/news/statements/2016/zika-third-ec/en/ (accessed July 7, 2016).

WORLD HEALTH ORGANIZATION. WHO statement on the first meeting of the International Health Regulations (2005) (IHR 2005) Emergency Committee on Zika virus and observed increase in neurological disorders and neonatal malformations. Geneva: World Health Organization, February 1, 2016e, www.who.int/mediacentre/news/statements/2016/1st-emergency-committee-zika/en/ (accessed July 7, 2016).

WORLD HEALTH ORGANIZATION. WHO public health advice regarding the Olympics and Zika virus. Geneva: World Health Organization, May 29, 2016f, www.who.int/mediacentre/news/releases/2016/zika-health-advice-olympics/en/ (accessed July 7, 2016).

WORLD HEALTH ORGANIZATION. Fifth meeting of the Emergency Committee under the International Health Regulations (2005) regarding microcephaly, other neurological disorders and Zika virus. Geneva: World Health Organization, November 18, 2016g, www.who.int/mediacentre/news/statements/2016/zika fifth-ec/en/ (accessed March 7, 2017).

WORLD HEALTH ORGANIZATION. *Zika situation report*: Zika virus, microcephaly and Guillain-Barré syndrome. Geneva: World Health Organization, February 2, 2017, http://apps.who.int/iris/bitstream/10665/254507/1/zikasitrep2Feb17-eng.pdf?ua=1 (accessed February 20, 2017).

# ABOUT THE AUTHOR AND TRANSLATOR

**Debora Diniz** is a professor of bioethics at the University of Brasilia. She also serves as a member of the Brazilian Ministry of Health's National Network of Specialists on Zika and Related Diseases, and as vice-chair of the International Women's Health Coalition (IWHC) board of directors. She is also an award-winning documentary filmmaker, and her most recent film, *Zika* (2016), draws on the experiences and research that informs this book.

**Diane Grosklaus Whitty** is a translator specializing in the fields of history, health, and the social sciences.